I0093738

PSYCHIATRY

in

PRIMARY CARE

PSYCHIATRY
in
PRIMARY CARE

A concise Canadian pocket guide

EDITED BY

David S. Goldbloom, MD, FRCPC

Jon Davine, MD, CCFP, FRCPC

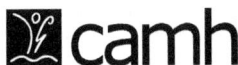

camh

Centre for Addiction and Mental Health
Centre de toxicomanie et de santé mentale

Library and Archives Canada Cataloguing in Publication

Psychiatry in primary care : a concise Canadian pocket guide / David S. Goldbloom,
Jon Davine, editors.

Includes bibliographical references and index.
Issued also in electronic format.
ISBN 978-0-88868-680-0

1. Psychiatry—Handbooks, manuals, etc. 2. Primary care (Medicine)—Handbooks, manuals,
etc. I. Goldbloom, David S II. Davine, Jon

RC454.4.P683 2011   616.89   C2011-900454-2

ISBN: 978-0-88868-680-0 (PRINT)
ISBN: 978-0-88868-681-7 (HTML)
ISBN: 978-0-88868-682-4 (PDF)
ISBN: 978-1-77052-663-1 (ePUB)

Printed in Canada
Copyright © 2011 Centre for Addiction and Mental Health

*No part of this work may be reproduced or transmitted in any form or by any means electronic or me-
chanical, including photocopying and recording, or by any information storage and retrieval system without
written permission from the publisher—except for a brief quotation (not to exceed 200 words) in a review
or professional work. Medicine is an evolving science. As new research and clinical experience broaden
our knowledge, changes in treatment are required. The authors and editors have referred to sources that
are believed to be reliable. The contents of this publication are based on information available as of 2011.
However, in view of the possibility of human error or changes in medical science, neither the authors,
editors, publishers nor any other party that has been involved in the preparation or publication of this
publication warrant that the information herein is in every respect accurate or complete, and they are not
responsible for any errors or omissions or for the results obtained from the use of such information. Readers
are encouraged to confirm the information contained herein with other sources.*

This publication may be available in other formats. For information about alternate formats
or other CAMH publications, or to place an order, please contact Sales and Distribution:

Toll-free: 1 800 661-1111
Toronto: 416 595-6059
E-mail: publications@camh.net

Online store: http://store.camh.net

Website: www.camh.net

This guide was produced by:
Development: Andrew Johnson and Susan Rosenstein (CAMH); Editorial: Kelly Coleman, Jacquelyn
Waller-Vintar (CAMH); Design: Mara Korkola (CAMH); Typesetter: Leonard Wyma, Donderdag;
Print production: Christine Harris (CAMH)

2973 / 09-2011 / PG126

Contents

Contributors

Susan E. Abbey, MD, FRCPC
Professor, Department of Psychiatry, University of Toronto; director, Program in Medical Psychiatry, University Health Network, Toronto, ON

J. Ellen Anderson, MD, MHSc
Assistant professor, Department of Family Practice, University of British Columbia, Vancouver, B.C.

Alexa Bagnell, MD, FRCPC
Assistant professor, Department of Psychiatry, Dalhousie University; associate chief of Child and Adolescent Psychiatry, IWK Health Centre, Maritime Psychiatry, Halifax, N.S.

Ash Bender, MD, FRCPC
Lecturer, Department of Psychiatry; medical director, Work, Stress and Health Program, Centre for Addiction and Mental Health, Toronto, ON

Dan Bilsker, PhD, R Psych
Adjunct professor, Faculty of Health Sciences, Simon Fraser University; clinical assistant professor, Faculty of Medicine, University of British Columbia Centre for Applied Research in Mental Health & Addiction, Simon Fraser University, Vancouver, B.C.

Marilyn A. Craven, MD, PhD, CCFP
Associate clinical professor, Department of Psychiatry and Behavioural Neurosciences, McMaster University, Hamilton, ON

Z. Jeff Daskalakis, MD, PhD, FRCPC
Associate professor, Department of Psychiatry, University of Toronto; staff psychiatrist, Schizophrenia Program, director of the Brain Stimulation

Treatment and Research Program, research section head for the Schizophrenia Program, Centre for Addiction and Mental Health, Toronto, ON

Jon Davine, MD, CCFP, FRCPC
Associate professor, Department of Psychiatry and Behavioural Neurosciences, with a cross appointment in the Family Medicine Department, McMaster University, Hamilton, ON

George Foussias, MSc, MD, FRCPC
Schizophrenia Program, Centre for Addiction and Mental Health, and Department of Psychiatry, University of Toronto, Toronto, ON

David S. Goldbloom, MD, FRCPC
Professor, Department of Psychiatry, University of Toronto; senior medical advisor, Education and Public Affairs, Centre for Addiction and Mental Health, Toronto, ON; vice-chair, Mental Health Commission of Canada

M.R. Goolam Hussain, MD, CCFP
Medical director, Tri-Hospital Sleep Laboratory West; Mississauga, ON

Umesh Jain, MD, FRCPC, PhD
Associate professor, Department of Psychiatry, University of Toronto; staff psychiatrist, Child, Youth and Family Program, Centre for Addiction and Mental Health, Toronto, ON

Nick Kates, MBBS, FRCPC
Professor, Department of Psychiatry and Behavioural Neurosciences, McMaster University; director of programs, Hamilton Family Health Teams, Hamilton, ON

Agnes Kwasnicka, MSc, MD, CCFP
Staff physician, Addiction Medicine Service, CAMH, Toronto, ON

Raymond W. Lam, MD, FRCPC
Professor and head, Division of Clinical Neuroscience, Department of Psychiatry, University of British Columbia; VGH and UBC Hospitals, Vancouver Coastal Health Research Institute, Vancouver, B.C.

Kenneth Le Clair, MD, FRCPC
Professor and chair of Geriatric Psychiatry, Queen's University; clinical director, Regional Geriatric Psychiatry Program, Providence Care, Mental Health Services, Kingston, ON

Paul S. Links, MD, FRCPC
Professor and Arthur Sommer Rotenberg Chair in Suicide Studies, Department of Psychiatry, University of Toronto; deputy chief of Mental Health Service, St. Michael's Hospital, Toronto, ON

Ellen Lipman, MSc, MD, FRCPC
Associate professor, Department of Psychiatry and Behavioural Neurosciences, Division of Child Psychiatry, McMaster University, Hamilton, ON

Roger S. McIntyre, MD, FRCPC
Associate professor of Psychiatry and Pharmacology, University of Toronto; head, Mood Disorders Psychopharmacology Unit, University Health Network, Toronto, ON

Brenda Mills
Clinician, Department of Psychiatry and Behavioural Neurosciences, McMaster University; co-ordinator, Child & Youth Mental Health, Hamilton Family Health Team, Hamilton, ON

Shaila Misri, MD, FRCPC
Clinical professor of Psychiatry and Obstetrics/Gynecology, University of British Columbia, Vancouver, B.C.

Gregor Novak, University of Ljubljana, Slovenia

Dallas Seitz, MD, FRCPC
Assistant professor, Geriatric Psychiatry, Queen's University; Providence Care, Mental Health Services, Kingston, ON

Peter Selby, MBBS, CCFP, MHSc, ASAM
Associate professor, Departments of Family and Community Medicine, Psychiatry and Public Health Sciences, University of Toronto; clinical director, Addictions Program and head of the Nicotine Dependence Clinic, and principal investigator, Ontario Tobacco Research Unit, Centre for Addiction and Mental Health, Toronto, ON

Colin Shapiro, MBBS, PhD, MRCPsych, FRCPC
Professor of Psychiatry and Ophthalmology, University of Toronto; director of the Sleep and Alertness Clinic and Sleep Research Laboratory, Toronto Western Hospital, Toronto, ON

Richard Swinson, MD, FRCPC
Professor emeritus, Department of Psychiatry and Behavioural Neurosciences, McMaster University, and Anxiety Treatment and Research Centre, St Joseph's Healthcare, Hamilton, ON

Dora Zalai, MD, Dipl. Psych
Counsellor, Sleep and Alertness Clinic, Toronto; International Sleep Clinic, Parry Sound, ON

Ari E. Zaretsky, MD, FRCPC
Associate professor and director, Postgraduate Education, Department of Psychiatry, University of Toronto; Centre for Addiction and Mental Health, Toronto, ON

Acknowledgments

The creation of this book was driven by the recognition that despite the fact that primary care clinicians provide the bulk of mental health care in Canada, no single Canadian book was targeted to meet their professional needs and ultimately the clinical needs of patients and families. We consulted an advisory panel of family physicians on the need for this book, as well as on the specific subject areas and even the chapter format. We are very grateful to them: Dr. Michael Evans, Dr. Allyn Walsh, Dr. Marilyn Craven, Dr. Chris Giles, Dr. Janet Wilson and Dr. Shawna Perlin. The planning for and production of this book was made immeasurably easier by the skilled support and wise counsel of our internal editors at CAMH, Andrew Johnson and Susan Rosenstein. And we are deeply appreciative of the contributions of our authors from across Canada, who shared our view that primary care physicians need a concise and practical guide for rapid diagnosis, intervention, education and support of Canadians with mental health problems and illnesses.

Introduction

DAVID S. GOLDBLOOM

Primary care health professionals know all too well that they are on the front lines in the provision of mental health care in Canada. At the same time, they are constrained by numerous factors in trying to recognize and meet the needs of their patients: time, knowledge, skills, supports and specialized referral access. In addition, the stigma that persists around mental illness can limit both patient disclosure and physician inquiry.

Psychiatry in Primary Care: A Concise Canadian Pocket Guide is intended to meet some of those needs in a practical and feasible way. It minimizes dry information about etiology and pathogenesis to focus on what primary care health professionals can ask, do, and recommend.

No guide can solve the problem of limited or no access to specialized care. However, new models for the delivery of psychiatric services are evolving rapidly, from shared care to televideo consultation (see the appendix for links to websites for shared care and telepsychiatry) that will overcome some of the geographic and wait list obstacles to collaborative care. Primary care health professionals should explore the availability of these kinds of resources in their community as they evolve.

The editors applaud the role of primary care professionals in meeting the mental health needs of Canadians and thank them for their efforts. We hope this handbook helps them in that important role.

1

The art of the brief psychiatric interview in primary care

JON DAVINE

In today's world, a significant part of being a primary care provider is dealing with people's mental health. It has been estimated that approximately 15 to 50 per cent of all patients encountered in the primary care ambulatory setting have emotional problems that are either primary in nature or secondary to physical illness. Many of these patients are seen exclusively in the primary care setting and, in fact, are not seen at all by mental health care specialists. This underlines the current and future importance of primary care in the delivery of mental health care to a community.

Primary care providers are in a wonderful position to get at these emotional issues due to the longitudinal nature of the relationship with their patients. Most people are seen in primary care on at least a yearly basis, and because of the ongoing nature of the relationship, and the trust that evolves, may be ready to share some of their emotional issues.

Unfortunately, detection rates of mental disorders in primary care remain low. There are a number of reasons for this. Firstly, there is usually very limited time available for each appointment. Also, patients who have emotional or psychiatric issues often present with a "somatic" presentation which may be seen as a valid "ticket of admission" instead of their emotional issues (see "The patient who is somatizing or is bodily preoccupied," page 61). Thirdly, there remains a stigma about psychiatric illness that may make patients more reluctant to discuss their issues.

Thus primary care providers are already delivering the bulk of mental health care to a community, though many mental disorders still remain undetected. This highlights the importance of the brief psychiatric interview in the primary care setting as a way to enable clinicians to "get at" psychiatric and psychological issues in a timely manner.

One of the most important things in terms of obtaining emotional information, which may be somewhat hidden, is simply "opening the door" by asking the patients screening questions. And don't ask with your hand on the doorknob at the end of the assessment! It has been shown, for example, that asking two simple questions—"over the past month, have you felt down, depressed or helpless?" and "over the past month, have you felt little interest or pleasure in doing things?"—can be helpful in the detection of depression. Obviously, if there are positive answers to these screens, then further questions on this topic can be asked.

Primary care providers should familiarize themselves with a number of specific screening questions that they can use for specific psychiatric disorders. Clearly, due to time constraints, the screening questions should be limited to those related to the specific problem(s) that the patient presents with on that day. They should be fairly stark, so that a positive answer would be quite significant, and should be pursued.

The following sections present a number of examples of possible screening questions for the different psychiatric disorders.

Screening questions for specific psychiatric disorders

Depression
· Have you ever had a period where you felt down? Not just for a week or two but, in fact, for many weeks and, perhaps, months?
· Did you find you had no energy, had no interest in things, and overall had great difficulty functioning?
· Has this ever happened to you before?

Hypomania/mania
· In the past, have you ever had a period where you felt not just good, but better than good?
· Did this feeling of unusually high energy and a decreased need for sleep go on not for hours or an evening but for days and days at a time?

Dysthymic disorder
· Have you felt down or low but able to function over the last number of years?

Generalized anxiety disorder
· Would you describe yourself as a chronic worrier? Would others say you are someone who is always worrying about things?
· Do you worry about anything and everything as opposed to just one or two things?
· If so, how long has this been going on?
· Some people tell me that they are worriers but they can usually handle it; other people tell me that they are such severe worriers that they find that worrying gets in the way of their life or simply paralyzes them. Is this the case for you?

Obsessive-compulsive disorder (OCD)

· Do you have any unusual or repetitive thoughts that you know are silly but you simply cannot stop yourself from thinking about (for example, being contaminated by germs)?
· Do you feel there are certain rituals you have to do, such as tap your hand a certain way or do things in sets of threes, which takes up a lot of time in the day?

Delusions and hallucinations

· Do you have unusual experiences such as hearing voices that other people cannot hear? What about seeing things that other people cannot see?
· Do you have unusual ideas, such as feeling that the TV or radio has special messages for you?
· Do you have unusual ideas that people you do not even know are plotting to harm you or kill you?
· Do you have unusual ideas, such as feeling that you have special powers that no one else has?

Panic attacks

· Do you have panic attacks or anxiety attacks? By that I mean an attack of anxiety that comes fairly suddenly and is rather uncomfortable and involves feeling a certain number of physical sensations such as heart palpitations, shortness of breath or dizziness.

Agoraphobia

· Do you avoid going certain places because you are fearful of having a panic attack? Has this feeling restricted your activities?

Posttraumatic stress disorder (PTSD)

· Do you find it hard to stop thinking about a very difficult event that has happened to you?
· Do you find that you have nightmares related to the event?
· Do you find that you have flashbacks—and by that I mean very vivid

daydreams or what we may call a "daymare" about the event?
· When something happens that reminds you of the event, does that trigger a very large response in you?
· Do you find that you avoid things that remind you of the event?
· Generally, do you feel anxious since the event and have trouble sleeping or startle easily?
· Do you feel that this event, and the way it has left you feeling, still gets in the way of your life?

Social phobia
· Are you able to go to social situations where you may have to interact with people you don't know well, or is that very daunting for you?
· Can you eat in restaurants in front of others?
· Were you able to give presentations in front of others when you were in school, or can you do it now?
· Do your social fears get in the way of your life?

Borderline personality disorder
· Do you feel you are still searching for your sense of who you are (self-identity)?
· By "sense of who you are" (self-identity), I mean do you have a set of values (what is important to you) that stays constant over time?
· Do you have long-term feelings of sadness?
· Do you have long-term feelings of anger?
· Do you find that your relationships usually get very difficult and end abruptly?
· Have you had thoughts of killing yourself on and off over the years?
· Have you tried to kill yourself in the past?
· Have you had episodes in the past where you tried to hurt yourself, not to kill yourself but simply to cause yourself pain or distract you from something?
· How do you feel after these episodes? (Patients often respond that they feel a sense of release or relief.)
· Do you often feel empty inside?

· Do you find that you can be feeling okay then suddenly feel angry or you can be feeling okay and suddenly feel sad? Does this happen a lot during the course of a day?
· Do you find that you do things on impulse and then regret it afterwards?

Interview tips

If someone comes in the office with somatic complaints that do not feel organic in origin but rather seem to be stress-based, there are a number of things to do to help make the mind–body link. Assure the patient that his or her complaints are "real" and "not all in your head." Assure your patient that you will do the necessary physical work-up to look at possible physical origins of these complaints but, at the same time, mention that emotional factors may also be a possible cause of the symptoms. You can use the examples of tension headache or butterflies in the stomach as illustrations of a pain that is "real" but is due to emotional rather than organic under-pinnings. This helps build a collaborative relationship with the somatizing patient, while still helping to shift into a mind–body paradigm.

You should ask about your patient's sexual life and past history of sexual abuse or sexual assault. The number of people who have been abused is distressingly high. Opening the door will be very important here as patients may not offer the information themselves, but once the door is opened, they may often tell some of the abusive events that have occurred in their lives. By asking these kinds of questions, you are giving the patient a "meta-message" about a number of things: you are saying that you are aware of these issues, that you are fine with opening up discussion about these issues, and that you are comfortable dealing with issues that may arise out of this discussion. This meta-message will help people open up to you.

Primary care providers may avoid bringing up certain topics, even though the topics are touched upon by the patient, because they may fear opening up a "Pandora's box" of issues. However, it is always useful to capitalize on openings patients naturally provide when they bring up important subjects themselves. It does not matter when in the interview this happens, either when the patient arrives or as the patient is leaving with his or her hand on the door. If something comes up near the end of an interview, a clinician can always underline its importance for the patient and bring the patient back for another interview in short order to continue the discussion. This "shelving" manoeuvre can be very useful in using patient initiative to obtain psychiatric data. Obviously, if very crucial information, such as suicidal ideation, comes out, this discussion cannot be put off and the interview will have to be extended.

Active listening

Practise "active listening." Watch the patient's body language and speech and label things directly with the patient. For example, a clinician may say, "I noticed you have been talking more quietly as you talk about your marriage." This may lead to further important information about the marriage. Summarize things back to the patient—this lets them know you have been listening and gives them a chance to correct any incorrect assumptions. Sometimes, simply repeating the last word a patient says may encourage him or her to say more.

For example:
Patient: "I have been having trouble recently with my mother-in-law."
Clinician: "Your mother-in-law?"

No matter how busy a clinician is feeling, it is essential to allow the patient time to speak. One study of internists showed that in 69 per cent of interviews, physicians interrupted their patients, on average, within the first 18 seconds of the encounter. These interruptions lead to inaccurate understandings of the patient's problems and incomplete data. Silence is golden and allowing the patient to speak for a minute or two will help useful information come out.

When patients speak freely, a lot of issues may be presented at the beginning of the interview. Though useful, this can be somewhat daunting for clinicians. A helpful mechanism for dealing with this is called "prioritizing and shelving." The clinician and the patient can prioritize the top one, two or three complaints to be dealt with that day. Other complaints can then be "shelved" as less urgent, and dealt with on another day. The patient can obviously help dictate what is prioritized, but certainly, if the clinician feels something is urgent, this can then be brought into the equation. This "meshing of agendas" often helps patients feel they are being listened to and their complaints validated.

If possible, having a flexible schedule that accommodates certain patients can be useful as well. For instance, if you know certain people are coming in to discuss emotional issues, you may schedule a slightly longer time for them, which may give you a little more latitude with these patients.

Taking a personal history

Taking a personal history can help primary care providers know the patient in a longitudinal way, which in turn helps them to better understand the themes permeating a patient's life. Though there is not the time to take a personal history with every patient, it is extremely useful for patients who are being actively treated for their current emotional or psychiatric issues. Table 1.1 presents a number of questions that can help you efficiently gather the essential information. They elicit important data that inform on the enduring emotional patterns of a patient's life. They also help illustrate where these patterns may have originated.

Primary care providers have an important role to play in the delivery of mental health care to a community. Patients will often disclose things to their family doctor that they may not to other physicians. By embracing the emotional/psychiatric side of medicine and making this a normal part of their patient interviews, primary care providers are making an invaluable service available to their patients. Clinicians can decide how far they want to follow these problems on their own, and when to refer to specialists. This can depend on the clinician's knowledge and confidence level with these issues. Our hope is that this book will help increase both of the above.

Table 1.1 Personal history

Where were you born and raised?

Was it a happy home or *not* such a happy home to grow up in? What made it not so happy?

Describe your mother (father). How did you get along with her (him) growing up and now?

How many siblings do you have? How did you get along with them growing up and now?

Were you ever physically abused growing up? Sexually abused?

How far did you go in school? How did it go academically? How did it go socially?

What has your work experience been like since school?

Can you tell me about significant romantic relationships you have had in your life?

Are you in a current relationship (marriage)? How is it going? If you have children, how is it going with them?

Do you have friends?

Who do you turn to for support?

In general, how do you feel about yourself?

In general, can you get close to people, or do you tend to keep a distance?

References

Beckman, H.B. & Frankel, R.M. (1984). The effect of physician behavior on the collection of data. *Annals of Internal Medicine, 101* (5), 692–696.

Regier, D.A., Goldberg, I.D. & Taube, C.A. (1978). De facto U.S. mental health services system: A public health perspective. *Archives of General Psychiatry, 35* (6), 685–693.

Clinical Situations

2

The patient who is depressed

RAYMOND W. LAM

Differential diagnosis

Organic conditions

Many medical illnesses can cause depressive symptoms, but they generally have other symptoms and signs associated with the primary disease.

Unless indicated by history and/or physical examination, screening blood tests need only include complete blood count and thyroid stimulating hormone test (to rule out anemia and thyroid disease).

Many medications and/or alcohol and substance use can present with depressive symptoms.

Grief and major psychosocial stressors (adjustment disorders)

Major depressive episode (MDE) can be differentiated from bereavement by severity of symptoms (e.g., psychosis or suicidality), presence of anhedonia (total loss of feelings of pleasure) and duration of impairment (longer than two months).

Adjustment disorders have subsyndromal number and severity of symptoms compared to MDE. Watchful waiting may be helpful to determine whether symptoms of adjustment disorder worsen or persist into a depressive episode.

Bipolar disorder
It is difficult to assess for hypomania because patients often do not recognize euphoric states as abnormal. Using a screening questionnaire is helpful.

Anxiety disorder
Depression is often secondary to, or comorbid with, many anxiety disorders, especially generalized anxiety disorder, social anxiety disorder and panic disorder.

Personality disorder (especially Cluster B)
Personality disorders usually present with lifelong patterns of mood instability.

How to make the diagnosis in less than five minutes (rapid assessment)
Use the two-question "quick screen" for patients with risk factors for MDE:
· In the past month, have you lost interest or pleasure in things you usually like to do? Have you felt sad, low, down, depressed or hopeless?
· An answer of "yes" to either question indicates the need for a more detailed assessment.

Risk factors for MDE include:
· chronic insomnia or fatigue
· unexplained somatic symptoms
· chronic medical illness
· recent cardiovascular event (myocardial infarction, stroke)
· recent trauma (psychological or physical)
· other psychiatric disorder

· family history of mood disorder
· extensive use of the medical system ("thick chart" syndrome).

Use a diagnostic questionnaire (e.g., the widely available patient-rated Patient Health Questionnaire [PHQ-9] for depression can be used for diagnosing, assessing severity of depression and monitoring response to treatment; see "Online resources" on page 24) along with the SIGECAPS mnemonic for symptoms of MDE (see page 15 for DSM criteria). SIGECAPS stands for:

· **S**leep (insomnia or hypersomnia)
· **I**nterest (reduced, with loss of pleasure)
· **G**uilt (often unrealistic)
· **E**nergy (mental and physical fatigue)
· **C**oncentration (distractibility, memory disturbance)
· **A**ppetite (decreased or increased)
· **P**sychomotor (retardation or agitation)
· **S**uicide (thoughts, plans, behaviours).

Use a screening questionnaire (e.g., the Mood Disorder Questionnaire) to rule out bipolar disorder.

DSM-IV-TR Criteria for Major Depressive Episode

A. Five (or more) of the following symptoms have been present during the same 2-week period and represent a change from previous functioning; at least one of the symptoms is either (1) depressed mood or (2) loss of interest or pleasure. **Note:** Do not include symptoms that are clearly due to a general medical condition, or mood-incongruent delusions or hallucinations.

   (1) depressed mood most of the day, nearly every day, as indicated by either subjective report (e.g., feels sad or empty) or observation made by others (e.g., appears tearful). **Note:** In children and adolescents, can be irritable mood

   (2) markedly diminished interest or pleasure in all, or almost all, activities most of the day, nearly every day (as indicated by either subjective account or observation made by others)

(3) significant weight loss when not dieting or weight gain (e.g., a change of more than 5% of body weight in a month), or decrease or increase in appetite nearly every day. **Note:** In children, consider failure to make expected weight gains

(4) insomnia or hypersomnia nearly every day

(5) psychomotor agitation or retardation nearly every day (observable by others, not merely subjective feelings of restlessness or being slowed down)

(6) fatigue or loss of energy nearly every day

(7) feelings of worthlessness or excessive or inappropriate guilt (which may be delusional) nearly every day (not merely self-reproach or guilt about being sick)

(8) diminished ability to think or concentrate, or indecisiveness, nearly every day (either by subjective account or as observed by others)

(9) recurrent thoughts of death (not just fear of dying), recurrent suicidal ideation without a specific plan, or a suicide attempt or a specific plan for committing suicide.

B. The symptoms do not meet criteria for a Mixed Episode.

C. The symptoms cause clinically significant distress or impairment in social, occupational, or other important areas of functioning.

D. The symptoms are not due to the direct physiological effects of a substance (e.g., a drug of abuse, a medication) or a general medical condition (e.g., hypothyroidism).

E. The symptoms are not better accounted for by Bereavement, i.e., after the loss of a loved one, the symptoms persist for longer than 2 months or are characterized by marked functional impairment, morbid preoccupation with worthlessness, suicidal ideation, psychotic symptoms, or psychomotor retardation.

Reprinted with permission from the *Diagnostic and Statistical Manual of Mental Disorders*, Fourth Edition, Text Revision (Copyright 2000). American Psychiatric Association.

Treatment options

Psychopharmacology

ACUTE TREATMENT
The goals for acute treatment of depression are full remission of symptoms and return to baseline function. Of depressed patients in primary care, 60 to 80 per cent can expect to achieve remission. Remission is defined as having normal mood and minimal symptoms, but is best evaluated using a rating scale (e.g., a score within the normal range on the PHQ-9, Hamilton Depression Rating Scale, Beck Depression Inventory). Antidepressant medications are first-choice treatments, especially for moderate to severe depression.

The newer antidepressants (selective serotonin reuptake inhibitors [SSRIs], bupropion, mirtazapine and venlafaxine) are all first-line medications, offering improved tolerability and safety profile compared to tricyclic antidepressants (TCAs) and monoamine oxidase inhibitors (MAOIs) (Tables 2.1 and 2.2 on pages 18 and 19).

Considerations when prescribing an antidepressant medication

Usually there is not one definite choice of medication for any given patient, since there is so much individual variability in efficacy and side-effects. Choice of antidepressant is based primarily on individual profiles of efficacy, tolerability and anxiety indications (Table 2.1 on page 18):

- There is some evidence for increased efficacy with escitalopram, mirtazapine and venlafaxine, particularly in patients with more severe depression.
- There is some evidence for better short-term tolerability with citalopram, escitalopram, moclobemide and sertraline. Bupropion, mirtazapine and moclobemide have fewer sexual side-effects than other antidepressants.
- A broad-spectrum agent (indicated for both depressive and anxiety disorders) is recommended due to high comorbidity of these disorders. Evidence for efficacy in most anxiety disorders is demonstrated with escitalopram, paroxetine, sertraline and venlafaxine. Other antidepressants *may* also be effective for anxiety disorders, but no studies have been done.

Table 2.1 First-line antidepressant medications, doses and profiles

FIRST-LINE ANTIDEPRESSANTS Generic name (brand name)	USUAL DAILY DOSE (mg)	EFFICACY[1]	TOLERABILITY[2]	ANXIETY[3]
SSRI				
citalopram (Celexa)	20–40		✓	
escitalopram (Cipralex)	10–20	✓	✓	✓
fluoxetine (Prozac)	20–40			
fluvoxamine (Luvox)	100–200			
paroxetine (Paxil)	20–40			✓
sertraline (Zoloft)	50–150	✓	✓	✓
SNRI				
desvenlafaxine (Pristiq)	50–100			
duloxetine (Cymbalta)	60–120	±		
venlafaxine-XR (Effexor)	75–225	✓		✓
Novel action				
bupropion-SR (Wellbutrin)	150–300	±		
mirtazapine (Remeron)	30–60	±		
trazodone (Desyrel)	200–400			
RIMA				
moclobemide (Manerix)	450–600		✓	

[1] Evidence for efficacy superiority based on meta-analyses and head-to-head trials.

[2] Evidence for better tolerability based on meta-analyses (Gartlehner et al., 2007).

[3] Evidence for efficacy in anxiety disorders based on Canadian guidelines (Canadian Anxiety Disorder Treatment Guidelines Initiative Steering Committee, 2006).

SSRI = selective serotonin reuptake inhibitor
SNRI = serotonin and norepinephrine reuptake inhibitor
RIMA = reversible monoamine oxidase inhibitor

Table 2.2 Second- and third-line antidepressant medications and doses

MEDICATION	USUAL DAILY DOSE (MG)
Second-line antidepressants	
TCA	
amitriptyline	100–250
clomipramine	100–250
desipramine	100–250
imipramine	100–250
nortriptyline	75–150
Third-line antidepressants	
MAOI*	
phenelzine	30–75
tranylcypromine	20–60

* Use with caution because of dietary restrictions and drug-drug interactions.

TCA = tricyclic antidepressant
MAOI = monoamine oxidase inhibitor

MAINTENANCE TREATMENT
The goal for maintenance treatment of depression is prevention of relapse and recurrence.
- Except for those with risk factors, patients should continue on antidepressants for at least four to six months after achieving remission.
- Patients with risk factors (chronic, recurrent, severe or difficult-to-treat depressive episodes) should continue on antidepressants for at least two years. Some will require lifetime treatment.

When stopping medications, gradually taper doses (e.g., at least one week for each dose reduction) whenever possible. Caution patients about, and monitor for, discontinuation symptoms (which are usually mild and transient). Discontinuation symptoms (mnemonic FINISH) include:

· Flu-like symptoms
· Insomnia
· Nausea
· Imbalance (dizziness)
· Sensory disturbances (electric shocks)
· Hyperarousal (agitation).

Discontinuation symptoms are more likely associated with paroxetine and venlafaxine, and are less likely with fluoxetine and moclobemide.

When there is *no* response to treatment, options include the following:
· Check diagnosis (any bipolarity, missed comorbidity such as substance abuse?).
· Optimize antidepressant: increase to maximum tolerable dose within dose range, ensure adherence for at least several weeks, manage side-effects.
· Add psychotherapy.
· Switch to another antidepressant: no difference between switching within the same class of first-line antidepressants (e.g., SSRI to another SSRI) or to a different class (SSRI to venlafaxine or bupropion).
· Augment with an augmenting agent. For example, add triiodothyronine (25 – 50 µg/d) or lithium (600 – 900 mg/d, or to therapeutic serum levels of 0.6 – 1.0 mmol/L). Alternatively, add an atypical antipsychotic (olanzapine 2.5 – 10 mg/d, risperidone 0.5 – 3 mg/d, quetiapine 100 – 300 mg/d). Be careful for increased side-effect burden, especially with lithium and atypical antipsychotics.
· Combine with another antidepressant in a different class. For example, add bupropion to SSRI. Be careful for drug-drug interactions and increased side-effect burden.

Although there is little evidence to guide decisions when there is only partial response to treatment, most clinicians would augment or combine in order not to lose gains from the first antidepressant.

A washout period usually is not necessary when switching between most antidepressants (*except* to and from MAOIs). Therefore, the second antidepressant can usually be started at low dose while tapering off the first antidepressant (the X approach). Be careful for increased side-effect burden when starting a medication before stopping another. In some patients, such as those who appear sensitive to side-effects, taper off the first antidepressant before starting the second (the V approach).

Avoid drug-drug interactions:
- Fluoxetine and paroxetine can markedly inhibit cytochrome P450 (CYP 450) isoenzyme 2D6 and can increase blood levels of drugs that are metabolized primarily by that isoenzyme (caution with TCAs, beta blockers, codeine [reduces effect]).
- Fluvoxamine can markedly inhibit CYP 1A2 and can increase blood levels of drugs that are metabolized primarily by that isoenzyme (caution with statin drugs, warfarin, quinidine, phenytoin, cyclosporine, sildenafil, vardenafil, clozapine, buspirone, diazepam).
- Duloxetine is extensively metabolized by CYP 1A2, so avoid using with potent inhibitors of CYP 1A2 (such as fluvoxamine and quinolones).
- MAOIs (and moclobemide) should not be combined with other antidepressants or serotonergic agents due to risk of potentially fatal interactions (e.g., meperidine).

Psychotherapy
In mild to moderate cases of depression, evidence-based psychotherapy is as effective as medication. Combining psychotherapy with medication does not work better than either alone except for patients with chronic, severe or refractory depression, or when comorbidity (anxiety, personality disorder) is present. The choice of psychotherapy depends on availability of local resources.

Evidence-based approaches include:
- Problem-solving therapy (PST): Four to six weekly sessions with a focus on identifying problems and simple problem-solving techniques, useful in primary care.
- Cognitive-behavioural therapy (CBT): 12 to 16 weekly sessions with a focus on identifying negative cognitions and behaviours, substituting more realistic thinking and behavioural activation.
- Interpersonal therapy (IPT): 14 to 16 weekly sessions with a focus on identifying and dealing with interpersonal conflicts and problems.

Self-management approaches should also be used (see next section).

Psychoeducation
Use simple messages to improve adherence to medications:
- "Antidepressants have a lag time of two to three weeks to response."
- "Take medications daily."
- "Side-effects are usually mild and temporary."
- "Continue on medications for at least six months, even after feeling better, or symptoms may return."
- "Do not stop antidepressants before checking with your doctor."

Self-management approaches
- Always include patient education (e.g., patient information handouts).
- Involve patients in the management of their own illness by actively collaborating with them in the diagnosis and treatment planning.
- Employ self-management manuals and workbooks (based on CBT techniques). See the list of resources on page 24.

Work and occupational function considerations
- This is an important aspect for treatment and psychosocial function.
- The patient may not need to take time off work. Balance benefits of staying at work (social interaction, regular schedule, sense of accomplishment) against risks (accidents, reduced productivity, interpersonal conflict).

· Address work stress using cognitive techniques and self-management. Note that avoiding stress is often counterproductive in dealing with depression.

Other treatments

Exercise and activity are beneficial for depression; therefore, "prescribe" at least one brisk walk daily. Light therapy (exposure to bright light using a fluorescent light box) is effective for seasonal affective disorder (recurrent winter depressive episodes). Electroconvulsive therapy is safe and effective for severe or medication-resistant depression. Electroconvulsive therapy should include psychiatric consultation and involvement.

What is reasonable to expect of a primary care clinician?

· Diagnose and develop a treatment plan.
· Assess suicide risk (see chapter 13, page 237).
· Monitor response and outcome using rating scales:
  - PHQ-9 is efficient because it is brief and patients can complete it at home or in the waiting room; it is also useful as a diagnostic aid and to identify remission status.
  - Full remission of symptoms is an important goal for acute and maintenance treatment.
· Coach self-management and/or use problem-solving therapy techniques.
· Manage medications:
  - Be familiar with at least two classes of antidepressants and at least one augmentation strategy.
· Refer when necessary (see next section).

When to refer to a specialist

· Complicating comorbidity (substance abuse, personality disorder, anxiety disorder)
· Severe presentation (serious suicidality, psychosis, bipolar disorder— especially Bipolar I, with manic episodes)
· Diagnostic clarification (bipolarity, personality disorder comorbidity)
· Refractory to standard treatment (CBT, two or more medication trials)

Community and online resources

Medical supports
· Community mental health clinics or hospital-based psychiatry outpatient clinics
· University- or hospital-affiliated mood disorders programs

Self-help or support groups
· Canadian Mental Health Association: www.cmha.ca
· Local mood disorders support groups, see Mood Disorders Society of Canada: www.mooddisorderscanada.ca

Self-management resources
· *Antidepressant Skills Workbook* by Dan Bilsker and Randy J. Paterson, BC Mental Health and Addiction Services, 2006 (72 pages). Available for free download at www.CARMHA.ca/publications.
· *The Feeling Good Handbook* by David D. Burns, Penguin Books, 1999.
· *Mind Over Mood* by David Greenberg and Christine Padesky, Guilford Press, 1995.

Online resources
· Canadian Network for Mood and Anxiety Treatments: www.canmat.org
· Canadian Mental Health Association: www.cmha.ca
· Mood Disorders Society of Canada: www.mooddisorderscanada.ca
· Mood Disorders Centre of Excellence: www.UBCmood.ca
· PHQ–9 questionnaires and instructions: www.depression-primarycare.org/clinicians/toolkits

References

Canadian Anxiety Disorder Treatment Guidelines Initiative Steering Committee, Swinson, R.P., Antony, M.M., Bleau, P., Chokka, P., Craven, M., Fallu, A. et al. (2006). Clinical practice guidelines: Management of anxiety disorders. *Canadian Journal of Psychiatry, 51* (8, Suppl. 2).

Gartlehner, G., Hansen, R.A., Thieda, P., DeVeaugh-Geiss, A.M., Gaynes, B.N., Krebs, E.E. et al. (2007). *Comparative Effectiveness of Second-Generation Antidepressants in the Pharmacologic Treatment of Adult Depression* (Comparative Effectiveness Reviews No. 7). Rockville MD: Agency for Healthcare Research and Quality.

Guidelines and Protocol Advisory Committee. (2004). *Depression (MDD): Diagnosis and Management.* Victoria, BC: British Columbia Ministry of Health. Retrieved from www.bcguidelines.ca/gpac/pdf/depression_full_guideline.pdf

Kennedy, S.H., Lam, R.W. & Morris, B. (2003). Clinical guidelines for depressive disorders: Summary of recommendations relevant to family physicians. *Canadian Family Physician, 49* (4), 489–491.

Kennedy, S.H., Lam, R.W., Nutt, D.J. & Thase, M. (2007). *Treating Depression Effectively: Applying Clinical Guidelines* (2nd ed.). London, England: Informa Healthcare.

Kroenke, K. & Spitzer, R.L. (2002). The PHQ-9: A new depression and diagnostic severity measure. *Psychiatric Annals, 32,* 509–521.

Virani, A.S., Bezchlibnyk-Butler, K.Z. & Jeffries J.J. & Procyshyn, R.M. (Eds.). (2006). *Clinical Handbook of Psychotropic Drugs* (18th rev. ed.). Toronto: Hogrefe & Huber Publishers.

3
The patient who is manic

ROGER MCINTYRE

Introduction

Bipolar disorder is a prevalent, progressive disorder associated with inter-episodic dysfunction and premature mortality. It is currently estimated that approximately 25 to 50 per cent of all individuals with depression in primary care settings have a bipolar spectrum disorder, one of the subtypes of bipolar disorder (Das et al., 2005). Nevertheless, under-recognition is common and protracted periods of time from the initial onset of affective symptoms to the correct establishment of the bipolar diagnosis are well documented. Most individuals with bipolar spectrum disorders presenting to both primary and specialty health care settings are mistakenly diagnosed as having a unipolar disorder. In keeping with this view, most individuals with bipolar spectrum disorders do not receive guideline-concordant care and, worse, receive inappropriate and possibly hazardous forms of treatment (antidepressant monotherapy) (McIntyre & Konarski, 2004).

Recent comorbidity studies indicate that most individuals with bipolar disorder are differentially affected by psychiatric and medical comorbidities. For example, anxiety disorders and substance use disorders are common co-occuring syndromes that frequently obscure the underlying mood disorder. The most common comorbid medical condition in bipolar disorder is overweight/obesity that often co-presents with other features of the metabolic syndrome (McIntyre et al., 2006). Taken together, comorbidity is associated with a greater illness severity, decreased response to treatment and, in the case of cardiovascular disease, premature mortality.

Primary care providers are in a unique position to screen, diagnose and treat bipolar spectrum disorders. Health service utilization studies indicate that people with bipolar disorder frequently use primary care services and employment assistance programs. The "illness burden" attributable to bipolar disorder is highly significant; it is now believed that bipolar disorder may be the most costly behavioural health disorder.

Differential diagnosis

Bipolar spectrum disorders

Bipolar spectrum disorders are categorized in the DSM into four types:
· Bipolar I Disorder (the presence of at least one manic or mixed episode)
· Bipolar II Disorder (hypomania and depression), possibly the most common bipolar presentation in primary care; affected individuals often use health services while depressed and often fail to respond sufficiently to conventional antidepressants (i.e., masquerade as treatment-resistant depression)
· Cyclothymic Disorder (continuous biphasic mood instability for two years or more in adults, but never severe enough to meet criteria for a major depressive episode or mania)
· Bipolar Disorder not otherwise specified.

As with all psychiatric disorders, the psychiatric disturbance should not be fully accounted for by the effects of a general medical condition or substance.

A common clinical scenario in primary care is a manic/hypomanic presentation in an individual receiving antidepressant monotherapy with no prior "de novo" manic or mixed episodes. Although the DSM classificatory schema would suggest these individuals are appropriately labelled as "antidepressant-induced," compelling evidence and growing expert consensus indicates that antidepressants do not engender mania but instead exacerbate pre-existing hypomanic symptoms and/or unmask hypomanic symptoms in a vulnerable individual. This is similar to gestational diabetes mellitus revealing an innate vulnerability to glucoregulatory disturbances.

Other considerations in differential diagnosis

Other considerations in the differential diagnosis of bipolar disorder include major depressive episode with prominent agitation/anxiety, premenstrual dysphoric disorder, seasonal affective disorder and characterological disorders (e.g., borderline personality disorder).

For example, borderline personality disorder is not a diagnosis of exclusion when detecting bipolar disorder. Many patients will have both conditions. The central and defining features of borderline personality disorder are an enduring and pervasive pattern of interpersonal relations that is chaotic and tempestuous, with subjective complaints of emptiness and "attachment difficulties." Individuals with borderline personality disorder often have distal trauma (e.g., childhood adversity).

Approximately 50 to 95 per cent of people with bipolar disorder will have psychotic features. Those affected are more likely to experience psychotic features during manic versus depressive episodes. Both mood-congruent (e.g., grandiosity) and mood-incongruent (e.g., paranoia) delusions are the most common psychotic features. Psychosis presenting as a form of thought disorder (e.g., tangentiality) is common. Although hallucinations and "vivid" perceptions are also common, the presence of hallucinations further underscores the need to rule out "organic" causes as well as substance use. In any person presenting with psychotic features, despite the presence of grandiosity and other mood-congruent features, the possibility of a primary psychotic disorder (e.g., schizophrenia) has to be considered in the differential diagnosis.

How to make the diagnosis in less than five minutes (rapid assessment)

In a primary care setting, a rapid assessment of a possibly manic/hypomanic patient needs to primarily address safety of the patient and family/caretakers as well as health care providers. The complexity and severity of symptoms in mania often necessitate hospitalization and the need for rapid and efficacious control of symptoms. Agitation, irritability and severe aggression are commonly encountered elements of mania and are associated with self-harm (Yatham et al., 2006; Yatham et al., 2009).

Primary care providers should consider routine screening for bipolar disorder in all patients who present with affective symptoms (Das et al., 2005). Individuals presenting with co-occuring anxiety disorders, substance use disorder or impulse dyscontrol (e.g., gambling disorders) should be closely scrutinized for clinical presentations suggestive of bipolar disorder.

In a busy office setting, the use of a screening tool such as the Mood Disorder Questionnaire (MDQ) is a valid and efficient way to probe for bipolar symptomatology (see "Online resources" on page 42). The MDQ is a patient-administered questionnaire with yes / no responses to 13 questions pertaining to experiencing manic / hypomanic symptoms. A positive screen is when patients answer "yes" to seven out of 13 of these questions, while also indicating that at least some of the symptoms are occurring concurrently and that they are causing a moderate level of functional impairment. A positive screen should be further questioned to confirm or refute a bipolar diagnosis (Hirschfeld et al., 2000).

Ruling out organic pathology

Organic pathology can be reasonably excluded by focusing on biological factors that may be associated with mania.

For example, a physical exam evaluating specifically for focal neurological signs and/or evidence of head trauma may be warranted. In addition, laboratory screening for thyroid abnormalities is generally recommended. It is also suggested that primary care providers consider and seek consent for toxicology screening if surreptitious illicit drug use is suspected.

Clinical clues to possible bipolar depression

The key elements of bipolar presentations in primary care include:
· the initial presentation of depression that progressed into treatment-resistant depression

· antidepressant monotherapy exacerbating/unmasking hypomania
· the prominence of anxiety, agitation and hyperactivity
· poor impulse control
· family history of mental illness
· early age onset of disturbance.

Treatment options

The treatment algorithm for bipolar mania is described in Figure 3.1. This was developed for psychiatrists treating bipolar mania and its latter steps are beyond the clinical practice of most primary care physicians.

The first task is to determine the treatment setting for the patient. Safety concerns related to self-harm and/or harm to others as well as neglect of personal care often provide the basis for immediate hospitalization.

The discontinuation of antidepressants is often a helpful first step in reducing manic severity. In most severe and complex presentations of mania, however, the removal of an antidepressant along with discontinuation of caffeine, alcohol and illicit substances is rarely sufficient on its own to bring about rapid symptom control. Many individuals experiencing mania are highly distressed by their behaviour as well as by the psychopathological symptoms (e.g., psychosis). You should provide empathic reassurance and attempt to engage the person in supportive ways. Offering education pertaining to the cause of the disturbance and discussing available treatment options are warranted.

Behavioural strategies include establishing normal daily rhythms with special emphasis on sleep hygiene and appropriate nutritional intake / hydration and energy expenditure.

Figure 3.1 Treatment algorithm for acute mania

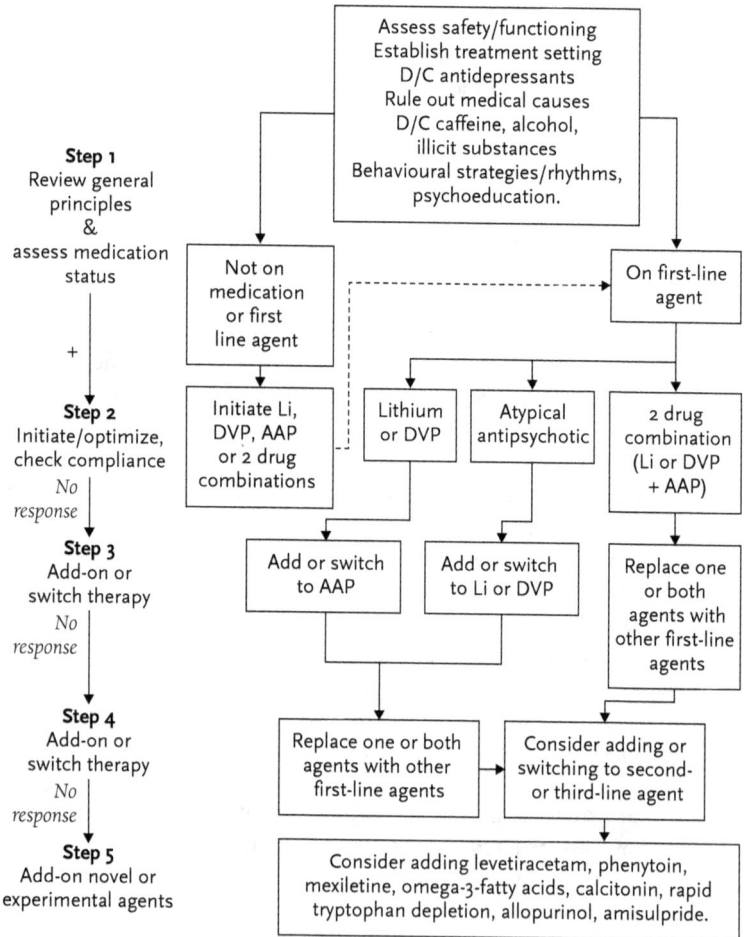

Step 1
Review general
principles
&
assess medication
status

+

Step 2
Initiate/optimize,
check compliance
*No
response*

Step 3
Add-on or
switch therapy
*No
response*

Step 4
Add-on or
switch therapy
*No
response*

Step 5
Add-on novel or
experimental agents

Assess safety/functioning
Establish treatment setting
D/C antidepressants
Rule out medical causes
D/C caffeine, alcohol,
illicit substances
Behavioural strategies/rhythms,
psychoeducation.

Not on
medication
or first
line agent

On first-line
agent

Initiate Li,
DVP, AAP
or 2 drug
combinations

Lithium
or DVP

Atypical
antipsychotic

2 drug
combination
(Li or DVP
+ AAP)

Add or switch
to AAP

Add or switch
to Li or DVP

Replace one
or both
agents with
other first-line
agents

Replace one or both
agents with other
first-line agents

Consider adding or
switching to second-
or third-line agent

Consider adding levetiracetam, phenytoin,
mexiletine, omega-3-fatty acids, calcitonin, rapid
tryptophan depletion, allopurinol, amisulpride.

D/C – discontinue; Li = lithium; DVP = divalproex; AAP=atypical antipsychotic

Reproduced with permission from Yatham et al., 2009.

Table 3.1 Recommendations for pharmacological treatment of acute mania

First line

Lithium, divalproex, olanzapine, risperidone, quetiapine, quetiapine XR, aripip-razole, ziprasidone, lithium or divalproex + risperidone, lithium or divalproex + quetiapine, lithium or divalproex + olanzapine, lithium or divalproex + aripiprazole

Second line

Carbamazepine, ECT, lithium + divalproex, asenapine, lithium or divalproex + asenapine, paliperidone monotherapy

Third line

Haloperidol, chlorpromazine, lithium or divalproex + haloperidol, lithium + carbamazepine, clozapine, oxcarbazepine, tamoxifen

Not recommended

Monotherapy with gabapentin, topiramate, lamotrigine, verapamil, tiagabine, risperidone + carbamazepine, olanzapine + carbamazepine

ECT = electroconvulsive therapy

Adapted with permission from Yatham et al., 2009.

Pharmacotherapy

The pharmacological treatment of an acute manic episode includes the use of lithium, divalproex sodium, and atypical antipsychotics alone or in combination (see Table 3.1). The decision to employ monotherapy or a combination of treatments is influenced by prior medication use as well as patient factors that may influence progress or safety. For an untreated individual presenting with mania, a first-line agent such as lithium, divalproex or an atypical antipsychotic as monotherapy can be considered. For patients who are insufficiently managed with monotherapy, switching to a separate antimanic monotherapy or combining antimanic treatments is recommended.

Table 3.2 Levels of evidence and clinical recommendations for treatment of bipolar disorder

TREATMENT	ACUTE MANIA LEVEL OF EVIDENCE (recommendation)	ACUTE DEPRESSION LEVEL OF EVIDENCE (recommendation)	PROPHYLAXIS LEVEL OF EVIDENCE (recommendation)
Lithium	I (A for mania, B for mixed)	I (A)	I (A)
Antiepileptic agents			
Divalproex	I (A for mania and mixed states)	III (B)	II (A)
Carbamazepine	I (C)	II (C)	II (C)
Lamotrigine	III (D)	I (A)	I (A)
Gabapentin	III (D)	III (D)	III (D)
Topiramate	III (D)	III (D)	III (D)
Oxcarbazepine	I (C)	III (D)	III (D)
Novel antipsychotic drugs			
Olanzapine	I (A)	I (B)	I (A)
Risperidone	I (A)	III (C)	II (B)
Quetiapine	I (A)	I (A)	III (C)
Ziprasidone	I (A)	III (D)	III (D)
Aripiprazole	I (A)	III (D/E)	I (A)
Novel antidepressants			
SSRIs, SNRIs, NaSSAs*	(E)	I (B)	III (D)

* SSRI = selective serotonin reuptake inhibitor; SNRI = serotonin noradrenaline reuptake inhibitor; NaSSA = noradrenaline specific serotinin antagonist

Mixed state is the simultaneous presence of mania and depression.

A – Recommended first-line treatment

B – Recommended second-line treatment

C – Recommended third-line treatment

D – No recommendation or proscription

E – Not recommended

Reprinted with permission from McIntyre et al., 2004. Copyright The College of Family Physicians of Canada, 2004.

LITHIUM

Lithium remains a highly efficacious pharmacological treatment for acute mania. For individuals presenting with "classic mania," which refers to the presence of euphoria, grandiosity and hyperactivity in a person with a stable episodic course, many experts would prefer lithium as a first-line agent. Most patients, however, presenting in clinical practice have more complex presentations that include, but are not limited to, dysphoric/mixed states (the simultaneous presence of mania and depression), comorbidity, psychotic features and rapid cycling (i.e., four or more affective episodes during the prior 12 months). In such complex presentations lithium may be less efficacious and the use of divalproex and atypical antipsychotics are preferred.

DIVALPROEX AND ATYPICAL ANTIPSYCHOTICS

Divalproex and atypical antipsychotics are highly effective in both classic and complex bipolar presentations. Since the early 2000s the atypical antipsychotic agents have been the most thoroughly studied agents for bipolar mania, offering efficacy not only in patients presenting with psychotic features but also in non-psychotic mania. Moreover, several atypical antipsychotics have also been established as efficacious in the treatment of acute bipolar depression and recurrence prevention as compared to other mood stabilizers (Perlis et al., 2006).

Table 3.3 Recommended agents and dosing in bipolar disorder

TREATMENT	DOSING	LABORATORY MEASURES	COMMON TREATMENT-EMERGENT ADVERSE EVENTS*
Antiepileptic agents			
Divalproex	Initiation: 500–1000 mg QHS; dosing based on 12 hrs trough plasma level (350–700 mmol/L)	Pre-treatment: CBC, electrolytes, TSH, liver function tests. Assure contraceptive being used (teratology risk); menstrual history required (i.e., DVPX associated with polycystic ovarian syndrome); repeat blood work including VPA level Q6 months if stable.	Sedation, somnolence, weight gain, menstrual irregularities, alopecia, tremor.
Lithium	Initiation 600–900 mg QHS; dosing based on 12 hrs trough plasma levels (0.8–1.2 meq/L; acute mania; 0.6–0.8 meq/L; maintenance/ depression)	Pre-treatment: CBC; electrolytes (including Ca++), TSH, BUN, creatinine. (EKG >40 yrs, or established heart disease/risk factors). Maintenance: lithium level: CBC; electrolytes (including Ca++), TSH, BUN, creatinine. Q6 months if stable. More frequently if symptomatic.	Sedation, cognitive dulling, weight gain, dermatological reactions (e.g., acne, eczema), polyurea, polydipsia, tremor.
Carbamaze-pine	Initiation: 600–900 mg; titrate as tolerated. 600–1200 mg.	Pre-treatment: same as above for divalproex; CBZ not associated with PCOS.	Sedation, somnolence, slurred speech, confusion, tremor.

Lamotrigine	Initiation: 25 mg Q2 weeks then 50 mg Q2 weeks followed by 100–300 mg daily.	CBC, electrolytes, no LTG levels required. Repeat Q6 months.	Headaches, gastrointestinal, dizziness, benign rash (10 per cent); serious rash (i.e., Stevens-Johnson syndrome; 1:1000).
Gabapentin	Initiation: 600–900 mg. Maintenance: 900–4000 mg in divided doses. Increase as tolerated Q2 weeks.	Same as lamotrigine.	Sedation, somnolence, confusion.
Topiramate	Initiation: 50 mg Maintenance: 100–300 mg. Titrate Q2 weeks as tolerated.	Same as lamotrigine. Include HCO3.	Cognitive dulling, word-finding diffi-culties, weight loss, metabolic acidosis, intensification of glaucoma.
Oxcarbaze-pine	Initiation: 150–300 mg. Maintenance: 300–1500 mg.	Same as carbamazepine.	Same as carbamazepine.

Novel antipsychotic drugs

Olanzapine	Initiation: 10–15 mg. Maintenance: 5–20 mg. Higher dosing in mania.	Pre-treatment: weight, BMI, fasting blood glucose, lipid frac-tionation, LFT, CBC, electrolytes. Repeat Q6 months. Repeat metabolic parameters more frequently in patients gaining weight.	Extrapyramidal symptoms (EPS), weight gain, dysgly-cemia, metabolic syndrome, seda-tion, somnolence, transient LFT elevation.

Table 3.3 Recommended agents, continued

TREATMENT	DOSING	LABORATORY MEASURES	COMMON TREATMENT-EMERGENT ADVERSE EVENTS*
Novel antipsychotic drugs, continued			
Risperidone	Initiation: 1–2 mg with a target of between 3 and 6 mg per day.	Same as olanzapine.	Same as olanzapine. LFT elevation not typically seen. Prolactin elevation/ prolactin-related side-effects.
Quetiapine	Initiation: 300–600 mg acute mania; 150–300 mg for acute depression; 150–450 mg maintenance in most patients. Titrate as tolerated (i.e., achieve recommended dose within 1–2 weeks); Quetiapine XR initiate 200 mg; increase to 300–600 mg in 2 days.	Same as olanzapine.	Same as olanzapine. LFT elevation not typically seen.
Ziprasidone	Initiation: 60–120 mg. Maintenance: 60–160 mg. Titrate as tolerated.	Same as olanzapine, EKG.	EPS, tremor, agitation, greater propensity to prolong QT interval. Akathesia, restlessness, minimal weight gain, metabolic disruption.

Aripiprazole	Initiation: 2.5 – 20 mg for acute. Maintenance: 2.5–30 mg. Titrate as tolerated.	Same as olanzapine.	Same as ziprasidone.
Novel antidepressants			
SSRIs, SNRIs, NaSSAs	Covered in antidepressant section. (See Table 2.1: "First-line antidepressant medications, doses and profiles" in chapter 2.)		Mobilization of hypo/mania and rapid cycling.

* No treatment for bipolar disorder is established as safe during pregnancy. Disparate teratogenetic effects are ascribed to each agent. Neural tube defects is the most replicated finding with divalproex and carbamazepine. Available safety data also suggest possible oral cleft defect with lamotrigine. Contraceptive methods with all bipolar treatments is recommended. In Canada, see Motherisk (www.motherisk.org/women/index.jsp) for more details regarding these and other agents.

A significant liability of most atypical antipsychotics is that they often cause significant weight gain and associated metabolic disruption. The probability of significant weight gain is further increased when these agents are prescribed with other weight-gain-promoting agents (e.g., lithium and some antidepressants). The decision to use a weight-gain-promoting atypical antipsychotic must take into consideration the benefits and probability of risk on an individual basis.

CONVENTIONAL ANTIPSYCHOTICS
Although historically conventional antipsychotics (e.g., haloperidol, perphenazine) have been frequently used in the treatment of bipolar disorder, these agents pose a hazard for both acute (e.g., akathisia, drug-induced Parkinsonism) and tardive (e.g., tardive dyskinesia) extrapyramidal side-effects. Clinical experience also suggests that conventional antipsychotics are

possibly associated with worsening of depressive symptoms in patients with bipolar disorder; as such, their use is discouraged (Zarate & Tohen, 2004).

BENZODIAZEPINES
Benzodiazepines are frequently prescribed to individuals with bipolar disorder and they are highly effective at reducing agitation, irritability and anxiety and normalizing sleep efficiency. In carefully selected cases, their use as adjunctive agents in acute situations is warranted. The possibility of non-therapeutic use of benzodiazepines in some patients with bipolar disorder, as well as "paradoxical" reactions in the form of worsening agitation, indicate that benzodiazepine use should be brief in duration and carefully monitored.

INITIATING PHARMACOTHERAPY AND ONGOING MANAGEMENT
It is generally recommended that if a patient is insufficiently responsive to antimanic monotherapy after one to two weeks, then an adjunctive treatment should be considered. If a patient stabilizes on combination therapy (e.g., divalproex and an atypical antipsychotic), and if the patient tolerates the treatment, it is recommended that the combination regimen be continued for a period of one to two years. If tolerability concerns (e.g., weight gain, menstrual irregularities) interfere with patient acceptance of either treatment, then consider engaging a psychiatric consultation as treatment moves into the continuation/maintenance phase.

Most primary care providers will initiate treatment for bipolar disorder while the patient is actively depressed. The selection and sequencing of treatment should be informed by the evidence presented in Table 3.2 and Table 3.3 (on pages 36–39). Antidepressant monotherapy is generally discouraged out of concern for destabilizing bipolar disorder. First-line pharmacological treatments for bipolar depression are lithium, lamotrigine or an atypical antipsychotic (e.g., quetiapine). In severe depression the use of an antidepressant in addition to the first-line agents (lithium, lamotrigine or an atypical antipsychotic) is suggested. For individuals who do not respond adequately to pharmacological treatments while depressed and/or presenting with severe symptomatology (e.g., psychotic symptoms) and/or functional impairments, electroconvulsive therapy should be considered.

Often a first-line mood stabilizer will be employed for the treatment of depressive symptoms in individuals ambiguously presenting as either major depression or Bipolar II. Opportunistic screening for clinical presentations suggestive of hypomania are warranted during long-term treatment. With the exception of lamotrigine, all available pharmacological treatments for bipolar disorder are more effective at forestalling or reducing the risk of recurrence of hypomania/mania than depression. In keeping with this view, pernicious subsyndromal (dysthymic/dysphoric) symptoms are a common clinical presentation despite adherence to pharmacotherapy and psychosocial treatment.

Tables 3.2 and 3.3 provide key information about the pharmacotherapies that may be considered for the treatment of bipolar disorder. Table 3.2 summarizes the levels of evidence supporting the use of medications both in terms of the problem being treated and their use as first-, second- or third-line medications. Table 3.3 provides an overview of available pharmacotherapies including information related to dosing, monitoring and side-effects.

What is reasonable to expect of a primary care clinician?

It is reasonable for a primary care provider to screen for and establish a diagnosis of bipolar disorder. Toward that aim, screening for secondary causes of mania is important. The ruling out of substance use disorder can be efficiently conducted through history and, if necessary, toxicology screening.

Providing psychoeducation and psychosocial/behavioural strategies is also warranted in primary care. Importantly, it is also reasonable for a family physician to begin treatment with antimanic pharmacotherapy.

When to refer to a specialist

If a specialty referral resource is available, a primary care provider
should refer to a specialist in any of the following scenarios:
- a patient requiring hospital admission
- questions regarding capacity for treatment decisions
- unfamiliarity with the use of anti-bipolar medications
- complex and uncertain clinical presentations
- diagnostic dilemmas
- cases of treatment-resistant mania
- problematic adverse events and safety concerns with medication
- when considering electroconvulsive therapy.

Community and online resources

- The Mood Disorders Psychopharmacology Unit, University Health
  Network, Toronto: www.mdpu.ca
- American Psychiatric Association: www.psych.org
- Canadian Network for Mood and Anxiety Treatments: www.canmat.org
- Canadian Psychiatric Association: www.cpa-apc.org
- Centre for Addiction and Mental Health: www.camh.net
- Depression and Bipolar Support Alliance: www.dbsalliance.org
- Health Canada: www.hc-sc.gc.ca
- Health Canada Drugs and Health Products: www.hc-sc.gc.ca/dhp-mps/
  prodpharma/index_e.html
- International Society for Bipolar Disorders: www.isbd.org
- *Moods Magazine*: www.moodsmag.com
- Mood Disorder Questionnaire and scoring instructions are on the Depression
  and Bipolar Support Alliance website: www.dbsalliance.org/pdfs
- National Alliance for Research on Schizophrenia and Depression:
  www.narsad.org
- The Mood Disorders Association of Ontario: www.mooddisorders.ca
- The Mood Disorders Society of Canada: www.mooddisorderscanada.ca.

References

Das, A.K., Olfson, M., Gameroff, M.J., Pilowsky, D.J., Blanco, C., Feder, A. et al. (2005). Screening for bipolar disorder in a primary care practice. *Journal of the American Medical Association, 293* (8), 956–963.

Hirschfeld, R.M., Williams, J.B., Spitzer, R.L., Calabrese, J.R., Flynn, L., Keck, P.E., Jr. et al. (2000). Development and validation of a screening instrument for bipolar spectrum disorder: The Mood Disorder Questionnaire. *American Journal of Psychiatry, 157* (11),1873–1875. DOI: 10.1176/appi. ajp.157.11.1873

McIntyre, R.S. & Konarski, J.Z. (2004). Bipolar disorder: A national health concern. *CNS Spectrums, 9* (11, Suppl. 12), 6–15.

McIntyre, R.S., Mancini, D.A., Lin, P. & Jordan, J. (2004). Treating bipolar disorder. Evidence-based guidelines for family medicine. *Canadian Family Physician, 50* (3), 388–394.

McIntyre, R.S., Konarski, J.Z., Wilkins, K., Soczynska, J.K. & Kennedy, S.H. (2006). Obesity in bipolar disorder and major depressive disorder: Results from a national community health survey on mental health and well-being. *Canadian Journal of Psychiatry, 51* (5), 274–280.

Perlis, R.H., Welge, J.A., Vornik, L.A., Hirschfeld, R.M. & Keck, P.E., Jr. (2006). Atypical antipsychotics in the treatment of mania: A meta-analysis of randomized, placebo-controlled trials. *Journal of Clinical Psychiatry, 67* (4), 509–516.

Yatham, L.N., Kennedy, S.H., Schaffer, A., Parikh, S.V., Beaulieu, S., O'Donovan, C. et al. (2009). Canadian Network for Mood and Anxiety Treatments (CANMAT) and International Society for Bipolar Disorders (ISBD) collaborative update of CANMAT guidelines for the management of patients with society bipolar disorder: Update 2009. *Bipolar Disorders, 11* (3), 225–255. DOI:10.1111/j.1399-5618.2009.00672.x

Yatham, L.N., Kennedy, S.H., O'Donovan, C., Parikh, S.V., MacQueen, G., McIntyre, R.S. et al. (2006). Canadian Network for Mood and Anxiety Treatments (CANMAT) guidelines for the management of patients with bipolar disorder: Update 2007. *Bipolar Disorders, 8* (6), 721–739.

Zarate, C.A., Jr. & Tohen, M. (2004). Double-blind comparison of the continued use of antipsychotic treatment versus its discontinuation in remitted manic patients. *American Journal of Psychiatry, 161* (1), 169–171.

4
The patient who is anxious

RICHARD SWINSON

Anxiety symptoms are extremely common. In the primary care setting a major task is to decide if the symptoms arise from a reaction to a distressing situation, are indicative of an anxiety disorder or another emotional disorder such as depression, or arise from an organic state.

Differential diagnosis

Adjustment disorder

Adjustment disorder is defined as a psychological response to an identifiable stressor, or stressors, that results in the development of clinically significant emotional or behavioural symptoms. These are short-duration conditions with symptoms developing within three months of the onset of the stressor and usually resolving within six months. An adjustment disorder with anxious mood is typified by nervousness, worry or jitteriness and in children by fear of separation from major figures (APA, 2000). The acute onset of anxiety symptoms following a major stressor such as marital separation, significant employment problems or threat to the stability of housing may all be followed by adjustment disorder with anxious mood. Screening for the disorders below (Table 4.1) is necessary to rule out the presence of anxiety, mood or organic disorders.

Organic states

Organic states such as hyperthyroidism can present with anxiety symptoms (e.g., tremulousness and palpitations). Is the clinical picture secondary to an organic state such as the intense agitation and fear in early stages of dementia? Is the use of stimulants (e.g., coffee, amphetamines) responsible for the occurrence of the symptoms?

Substance use disorders

People with anxiety may seek quick relief from commonly available substances. Is the withdrawal of benzodiazepines or alcohol responsible for the occurrence of the symptoms? It is important to ask in every case. There are both young and elderly patients who calm themselves with over-the-counter agents.

In addition, the use of stimulants can trigger significant anxiety symptoms and panic attacks. Three or four coffees, teas or caffeinated soft drinks daily can precipitate anxiety attacks. Cocaine and amphetamines are also powerful anxiety-producing agents. Although marijuana use is usually accompanied by feelings of relaxation, some people are very sensitive to the occurrence of depersonalization and suffer marked panic usually on one of the first few occasions that they try it.

Mood disorders

Depression often presents with anxiety symptoms that may be new or may be an exacerbation of pre-existing anxiety conditions that only come to attention as the mood state worsens. The combination of depression and severe anxiety symptoms is cause for concern due to an increase in suicidality. (See chapter 2, "The patient who is depressed," for screening methods for mood disorders.)

Personality disorders

Life-long mood instability as seen in Cluster B (borderline, histrionic and narcissistic) personality disorders may present with severe anxiety symptoms at times of increased instability.

Table 4.1 Brief diagnostic criteria for anxiety disorders

DISORDER	MAIN SYMPTOMS
Panic disorder with or without agoraphobia (PDAG)	Sudden, severe repeated attacks of anxiety some of which are "out of the blue." Fear of physical symptoms. May be avoidance of feared situations.
Agoraphobia without panic	Avoidance of feared situations (e.g., enclosed spaces, crowds, being away from home) without a history of panic attacks.
Specific phobia (SP)	Fear and avoidance of specific objects/places (e.g., snakes, dogs, sight of blood, heights, storms, tunnels, flying).
Social anxiety disorder (SAD)	Fear and avoidance of public performance or situations of being judged. May be limited or generalized to almost all social interactions.
Obsessive-compulsive disorder (OCD)	Unwanted, uncontrollable, repetitive thoughts (obsessions) and repetitive neutralizing actions (compulsions).
Posttraumatic stress disorder (PTSD)	Re-experiencing of a severe traumatic event through dreams, flashbacks and intense emotion with increased arousal and avoidance of reminders of the trauma.
Acute stress disorder (ASD)	Symptoms similar to PTSD occurring immediately after an extremely traumatic event.
Generalized anxiety disorder (GAD)	Persistent, uncontrollable worry lasting at least six months.
Anxiety disorder due to general medical condition	Symptoms of anxiety that are a direct physiological consequence of a general medical condition.
Substance-induced anxiety disorder	Symptoms of anxiety that are a direct physiological consequence of a drug of abuse, a medication or toxin exposure.
Anxiety disorder not otherwise specified	Anxiety symptoms not meeting the criteria for any of the specific disorders above.

Differential diagnosis within the anxiety disorders

The anxiety disorders are classified into eight "primary" disorders and two "induced" disorders. Common features include:

- physical symptoms of anxiety (e.g., tension, restlessness, GI symptoms)
- cognitive symptoms (e.g., fear, apprehension and worry)
- behavioural symptoms (avoidance and escape).

The specific anxiety disorders summarized in Table 4.1 are differentiated from one another by the prominence of particular symptoms.

Screening for anxiety disorders

When anxiety is a presenting symptom, screen to determine the specific anxiety disorder present, if any. Diagnosis of an anxiety disorder requires that the symptoms are the cause of significant distress or impairment in function.

Panic disorder (PD)

Ask the patient about:

- sudden unexpected episodes with a rush of symptoms or uncomfortable feelings such as racing heart or dizziness accompanied by feelings of panic or fear
- avoidance or hesitation to approach situations expected to bring on the symptoms (e.g., crowds, enclosed spaces, driving or leaving the house alone).

Panic disorder is frequently accompanied by avoidance of places where attacks have occurred or where the person fears that they might occur. This is called agoraphobia.

Agoraphobia (without panic)

Ask the patient about:

- avoidance of, for example, crowds, lines, bridges, going outside the home alone, travelling on bus, train or highway, or the need to have a companion as a safe person.

Note that complete houseboundedness is rare but is a strongly negative prognostic factor.

Social anxiety disorder (SAD)

This common anxiety disorder is characterized by fear of embarrassment or of negative evaluation by other people. It usually has very early onset and commonly begins in childhood or adolescence. People with SAD are frequently embarrassed about the condition and do not readily volunteer information about their anxieties.

Ask the patient: "In general, are you overly anxious or concerned about embarrassing or humiliating yourself while doing things in front of people or interacting with others?"

The severity of SAD can be assessed by asking three questions that make up the Mini-SPIN (Connor et al., 2001).

Mini-SPIN

Please choose the answer that best describes how much the following problems have bothered you during the past week. Circle a number for each problem and be sure to answer all the items.

	Not at all	A little bit	Somewhat	Very much	Extremely
	0	1	2	3	4
1. Fear of embarrassment causes me to avoid doing things or speaking to people.	0	1	2	3	4
2. I avoid activities in which I am the center of attention.	0	1	2	3	4
3. Being embarrassed or looking stupid are among my worst fears.	0	1	2	3	4

A score of 6 or greater is considered to strongly suggest the presence of Social Anxiety Disorder and indicates the need for further clinical assessment to rule the disorder in or out.

Reprinted with permission. Copyright Jonathan Davidson, 1995, 2010. The Mini-SPIN may not be copied, altered or distributed without permission.

Specific phobia (SP)

Specific phobias are the most prevalent anxiety disorders. They are usually not diagnosed because people learn to manage their anxiety by avoidance. Specific phobias can be very disabling if they involve situations that cannot be avoided such as having to attend a physician's office where blood tests may be ordered or needing to take an elevator to the 25th floor to get to work.

Ask the patient:
· Do any of the following make you anxious or fearful:
  - animals, snakes, insects
  - heights, storms, being near water
  - the sight of blood, getting an injection
  - being in enclosed spaces, flying, elevators?
· Does this fear interfere with your life?

Obsessive-compulsive disorder (OCD)

OCD is a disorder with onset as early as age four or five. It is frequently concealed by those who have it. The thoughts and impulses are recognized as unrealistic but are accompanied by shame at the content of, and the inability to control, the thoughts. There is intense compulsion to continue the thoughts and rituals and severe distress if they are resisted. This contrasts with "addictive" behaviours that produce pleasure or gratification.
· Ask the patient: "Do you experience repeated unwanted thoughts that you cannot easily control?" "Do you feel compelled to carry out repetitive acts, such as washing, counting or checking?"
· Symptoms of OCD include washing, checking, counting, hoarding, reassurance seeking and religious preoccupation.

Generalized anxiety disorder (GAD)

GAD is very common and occurs throughout the lifespan. The main symptoms are excessive, uncontrollable worry accompanied by muscle tension, fatigue, insomnia, impaired concentration and irritability. It is frequently comorbid with major depression.

- Ask the patient: "During the past four weeks, have you been bothered by feeling worried, tense or anxious most of the time?" Of people with GAD, 90 per cent will respond "yes" to this question.
- If positive, explore further symptoms. The WHAT IF mnemonic is useful:
  - **W**orry
  - **H**ard-to-control headache
  - **A**nxiety
  - **T**ension
  - **I**nsomnia/irritability/irritable bowel
  - **F**atigue.

Posttraumatic stress disorder (PTSD)

PTSD is precipitated by severe trauma in which the patient experienced, saw or heard of someone's physical or mental integrity being threatened. Feelings of horror and helplessness often occur at the time of the trauma. The onset of symptoms maybe delayed by months or even years and is triggered by another traumatic episode. The memories of the trauma remain very clear and are accompanied by intense emotion.

- Ask the patient: "Are you bothered by memories, thoughts or images of a very upsetting event that happened to you or to someone close to you in the past?" Offer examples such as being in a fire, accident, rape or seeing someone badly injured.

Underlying organic pathology

The necessary investigations depend on the patient's clinical presentation, age, sex, previous health history and other individual and familial factors. The Canadian Anxiety Disorders Treatment Guidelines suggest the following as a guide to screening an anxious patient (Canadian Anxiety Disorder Treatment Guidelines Initiative Steering Committee, 2006).

BASELINE LABORATORY INVESTIGATIONS IN PATIENTS WITH
ANXIETY DISORDERS
· Complete blood count
· Urinalysis
· Fasting glucose
· Fasting lipid profile (total cholesterol, very low density lipoprotein,
  low density lipoprotein, high density lipoprotein, triglycerides)
· 24-hour creatinine clearance (if history of renal disease)
· Electrolytes
· Thyroid-stimulating hormone
· Liver enzymes
· Electrocardiogram (if over 40 years of age or if indicated)
· Serum bilirubin
· Pregnancy test (if relevant)
· Serum creatinine
· Prolactin
· Urine drug screening for substance use (see page 94)

Treatment options

All patients should receive education including information about their
disorder, the available treatment choices and where they can obtain reliable
self-help material.

Both psychopharmacological and psychotherapeutic treatments provide
high response rates for all the anxiety disorders. Specific phobias rarely
need medication and should be treated with psychological interventions.

Acute treatment

Treatment choice depends on the acuity and severity of the presenting
condition. In most cases the symptoms have been present for months or
years before patients seek treatment.

Where there is a severe onset or exacerbation of an anxiety disorder with marked impairment of functioning and there is no contraindication, the benzodiazepines remain a very effective *short-term* option. In PTSD there is no observed benefit from administering benzodiazepines acutely.

In the absence of a crisis, initial treatment includes reducing and excluding all caffeine and alcohol. Give information about the most probable anxiety disorder present. Self-help techniques from books and trusted websites are indicated initially. Review in two weeks. If the anxiety continues and time is available, use self-help material in guided self-help (see chapter 20, "Supported self-management for common mental health problems," page 351).

If progress is made, continue with self-help. If not, discuss medication or cognitive-behavioural therapy (CBT). If the patient selects CBT, advise continuation with self-help using a CBT-based book and look for a referral source.

Overview of pharmacological treatment

Medications are the most frequently delivered treatment for anxiety disorders (see Table 4.2 on page 56 for first-line antidepressant medications, indications, doses and cautions). They are accessible and readily used by those who choose to take them. They can be costly and they all have side-effects.

Medications with evidence to support their use in anxiety fall into three groups. These are antidepressants, anxiolytics and other psychotropic agents used mainly to augment antidepressants.

ANTIDEPRESSANTS

All of the antidepressants have been shown to be variously effective in reducing the symptoms of the anxiety disorders. The SSRIs and SNRIs have repeatedly been found to be effective in treating panic disorder, social anxiety disorder, obsessive-compulsive disorder, posttraumatic stress disorder and generalized anxiety disorder (Table 4.2). There is also evidence for the efficacy for NaSSAs. The TCAs and MAOI/RIMAs are effective but are generally less well tolerated than SSRI/SNRIs and are reserved for later choice.

All antidepressants should be started at a very low dose in anxiety disorders. Anxious patients can be extremely intolerant of the side-effects of agitation and akathisia that may occur at the onset of treatment. Doses of fluoxetine and escitalopram as low as 5 mg daily are often necessary. Use the lowest dose available of SNRIs (e.g., venlafaxine 37.5 mg daily). Despite starting at a low dose, the ultimate effective dose is usually the same as in major depression or even higher. Anxiety disorders commonly need prolonged treatment before the desired results are achieved. It is better to start at a low dose with gradual increase over a long period of time than it is to challenge patients with doses that they cannot tolerate, leading to frequent switching of medications.

If the first SSRI/SNRI does not help at all after eight weeks, then discontinue (also slowly) and substitute another SSRI/SNRI. If two medications do not produce benefit consider referral for specialist opinion. In OCD, consider a switch to clomipramine with the usual precautions for tricyclics (e.g., cardiac arrhythmias, seizure risk and suicide risk). If there is partial benefit, consider augmentation by adding another agent.

The overall length of medication treatment in anxiety disorders is commonly 12 months or more followed by slow tapering. Many patients will relapse during the withdrawal phase. The rate of relapse is reduced when treatment includes CBT while medication is administered, or when it is introduced at the time of tapering the dose.

ANXIOLYTICS
Benzodiazepines are effective in most anxiety disorders. They do not offer much benefit in OCD. Care needs to be taken in PTSD due to very high rates of comorbid substance use disorders. It is advisable to avoid benzodiazepines in acute stress disorder.

Dependence is a significant problem. Inter-dose exacerbation of anxiety can be confused with worsening of the original disorder. When benzodiazepines are used, it is advisable to have a contract with the patient about the discontinuation date. Six to eight weeks of use in a new case is the suggested limit while an antidepressant is co-administered and then continued as the benzodiazepines are tapered.

Buspirone can be helpful in GAD and to augment antidepressant treatment. It does not have the acute therapeutic effects of benzodiazepines.

AUGMENTATION STRATEGIES

Many agents can be used to attempt to enhance the effects of antidepressants in all the anxiety disorders. Atypical antipsychotics have been shown to add to the improvement with antidepressant treatment. In OCD, the evidence is well established for the addition of haloperidol or risperidone in low dosage (0.5 mg daily or twice a day) to SSRI/SNRI. The combination is particularly effective in the presence of tics (McDougle et al., 1994).

In comorbid cases where an anxiety disorder occurs with a second disorder, augmenting the anti-anxiety treatment with a drug for treating the second disorder can be very useful (e.g., SSRI/SNRI plus anticonvulsant in anxiety disorder with bipolar disorder; SSRI/SNRI plus stimulant for comorbid ADHD).

Atypical antipsychotics have been extensively studied as monotherapy in anxiety disorders. They are not currently approved for this indication in Canada.

Psychotherapy

For treating anxiety, cognitive-behavioural therapy (CBT) is the psychotherapy with the best evidence base and therefore is the first-line psychotherapy. Depending on an individual's response to CBT, the severity and complexity of any comorbidity, and possible personality problems, other types of psychotherapy may be indicated. Patient choice is an important factor in the success of any therapy for anxiety. Those who choose CBT generally do better than those who are assigned to it without choice. When CBT is instituted, an adequate treatment trial should be administered, with appropriate monitoring and long-term follow-up.

Table 4.2 First- and second-line antidepressant medications, indications, doses and cautions

MEDICATION	INDICATIONS*	USUAL DAILY DOSE (MG)	CAUTIONS
First-line antidepressants			
SSRI			
Citalopram (Celexa)	PD	20–40	Initial agitation, worsening of panic attacks, increased suicidal ideation in young patients (<25 years). Weight gain, sexual problems.
Escitalopram (Cipralex)	GAD, OCD, PD	5–40	
Fluoxetine (Prozac)	OCD, PD, PTSD	5–60	
Fluvoxamine (Luvox)	OCD, PD, SAD	50–250	
Paroxetine (Paxil)	GAD, OCD, PD, PTSD, SAD	10–50	
Sertraline (Zoloft)	GAD, OCD, PD, PTSD, SAD	50–200	
SNRI			
Duloxetine (Cymbalta)	GAD	60–120	As above.
Venlafaxine XR (Effexor)	GAD, PD, PTSD, SAD	37.5–225	
Second-line antidepressants			
TCAs			
Imipramine	PD	25–150	Cardiac toxicity, overdose effects. Seizure risk at higher doses.
Clomipramine	OCD, PD	25–150	
Novel action			
Bupropion-SR (Wellbutrin)	Augmentation	150–300	Agitation.
Mirtazapine (Remeron)	Augmentation	30–60	Sedation, weight gain.

RIMA/MAOI

Moclobemide (Manerix)	SAD	300–900	Dietary restrictions
Tranylcypromine (Parnate)	OCD (third line)	20–60	at all doses for
			tranylcypromine
			and higher doses
			for moclobemide.

*Canadian Anxiety Disorder Treatment Guidelines Initiative Steering Committee, 2006.

Minimal exposure-based CBT can be effective. A very brief resource for practitioners is included in the Canadian Anxiety Disorders Treatment Guidelines (Canadian Anxiety Disorder Treatment Guidelines Initiative Steering Committee, 2006).

CBT is effective in individual and in group formats and overall CBT is as effective as drug therapy. There is no evidence that routinely combining medication and CBT is more effective than either treatment alone. When CBT is used, the patient's progress is monitored session by session. If insufficient progress is made, therapy can be modified to fit the specific patient's needs rather than switching to another psychotherapy. The amount of time allotted and the frequency of CBT sessions are important. Ideally two sessions a week of 60 or 90 minutes should be provided. Twelve to 20 sessions, depending on the disorder, will usually be sufficient to produce therapeutic effect. Follow-up sessions at monthly intervals are useful in maintaining gains. These can occur in self-help community-based groups.

What is reasonable to expect of a primary care clinician?
· Follow up on complaints of anxiety.
· Clarify the major anxiety symptoms, use screening questions.
· Discuss probable diagnosis.
· Offer psychoeducation about self-help, psychotherapy, medication use.
· Refer for community-based self-help if available.

- If time and resources are available, provide:
  - bibliotherapy
  - self-help with assistance
  - brief exposure-based treatment
  - more intensive treatment if trained counsellors are available in the practice setting.
- Offer medication treatment:
  - SSRI or SNRI +/- BZD
  - second SSRI or SNRI
  - specific augmentation.

When to refer to a specialist

- Following an attempt to treat the patient or earlier if the patient is significantly impaired
- With anxious children/adolescents who are too fearful to attend school or to socialize.
- With adults who cannot get to work or maintain their usual activities of daily living (e.g., child care, going shopping, hygiene)
- In the presence of multiple comorbid mental disorders (e.g., depression, substance use, suicidality)

Community and online resources

- Medical supports such as community-based mental health clinics or hospital psychiatry outpatient clinics, and specialty university-affiliated anxiety disorders clinics
- Other professional services
- Private psychological services

Self-help or support groups

- Canadian Mental Health Association: www.cmha.ca
- Local anxiety disorders support groups, see the Anxiety Disorders Association of Canada: www.anxietycanada.ca

· Provincial resources, for example, Anxiety BC (www.anxietybc.com), Anxiety Disorders Association of Manitoba (www.adam.mb.ca)

Self-management resources
· Links to disorder-specific resources are available at the Anxiety Treatment and Research Centre, St. Joseph's Hospital, Hamilton, Ontario: www.anxiety treatment.ca

Websites
· Anxiety Disorders Association of America (www.adaa.org). This is the largest international patient-centred anxiety organization and has high-quality, up-to-date information.
· The OCD Foundation (www.ocfoundation.org). This foundation provides information specifically for OCD and related disorders.

References

Antony, M.M. & Norton, P. (2008). *The Anti-Anxiety Workbook: Proven Strategies to Overcome Worry, Phobias, Panic, and Obsessions*. New York: Guilford Press.

American Psychiatric Association. (2000). *Diagnostic and Statistical Manual of Mental Disorders* (4th ed., text rev.). Washington, DC: Author.

Canadian Anxiety Disorder Treatment Guidelines Initiative Steering Committee, Swinson, R. P., Antony, M.M., Bleau, P., Chokka, P., Craven, M., Fallu, A. et al. (2006). Clinical practice guidelines: Management of anxiety disorders. *Canadian Journal of Psychiatry, 51* (8, Suppl. 2).

Connor, K.M., Kobak, K.A., Churchill, L.E., Katzelnick, D. and Davidson, J.R.T. (2001). Mini-SPIN: A brief screening assessment for generalized social anxiety disorder. *Depression and Anxiety, 14* (2), 137–140. DOI: 10.1002/da.1055

McDougle, C.J., Goodman, W.K. & Leckman, J.F. (1994). Haloperidol addition in fluvoxamine-refractory obsessive-compulsive disorder: A double-blind, placebo-controlled study in patients with and without tics. *Archives of General Psychiatry, 51*, 302–308.

Swinson, R.P. (2007). Anxiety disorders. In J. Gray (Ed.), *Therapeutic Choices* (5th ed.; pp. 11–26). Ottawa: Canadian Pharmacists Association.

5

The patient who is somatizing or is bodily preoccupied

SUSAN E. ABBEY

In every primary care clinic there are challenging patients who are preoccupied with bodily complaints, or with the fear of disease, despite no apparent medical basis for these concerns. Unless one has an effective approach to their management, these patients are both difficult and unsatisfying to treat because of the amount of time that they can take up and the general lack of satisfaction associated with their care. While these patients have many complaints, by definition they do not have a "lesion" that we can diagnose and treat.

Useful concepts to help us think about the patient who is bodily preoccupied

Somatization

Somatization is a concept that despite its long and convoluted history has come under considerable critique in recent years. Early in the 20th century, somatization referred to bodily symptoms thought to result from unconscious neurotic conflict. Since the 1980s, it has been used to describe patients who have a tendency to experience and communicate psychological and interpersonal distress in the form of physical symptoms or suffering, and to seek help for these symptoms.

Medically unexplained symptoms (MUS)

Currently, "medically unexplained symptoms" is the most widely used term for symptoms that are the focus of clinical attention and which disrupt quality of life, but for which a biomedical explanation cannot be found. Functional somatic syndrome is another term used to refer to these symptoms.

FUNCTIONAL SOMATIC SYNDROMES

Functional somatic syndromes are syndromes for which a clear pathophysiology has not yet been described and which are characterized by the reporting of MUS and disability rather than consensually agreed upon evidence of an underlying disease process (e.g., irritable bowel syndrome, non-cardiac chest pain, chronic fatigue syndrome, atypical facial pain, chronic pelvic pain, multiple chemical sensitivity, etc.).

The value of making these diagnoses is the subject of debate. It may be helpful in "ending the search" for a diagnosis. Yet in providing a diagnosis, we should emphasize the possibility of active management that increases function and quality of life.

Somatoform disorders

Somatoform disorders are a DSM-IV-TR diagnostic category. It is a category that includes seven disorders presenting with physical symptoms that cause significant distress or impairment in daily functioning that might otherwise suggest a medical condition and yet are not fully explained by a general medical condition, substance use or another psychiatric disorder. The seven disorders are:

· Somatization Disorder
· Undifferentiated Somatoform Disorder
· Conversion Disorder
· Pain Disorder
· Hypochondriasis
· Body Dysmorphic Disorder
· Somatoform Disorder not otherwise specified (American Psychiatric Association, 2000).

Differential diagnosis

The patient who is somatizing has a wide potential for differential diagnosis. The likelihood of a given diagnosis in an individual patient varies considerably. On a population basis, the common diagnoses follow, in order of likelihood.

Undiagnosed major psychiatric disorder

Over half of patients with a major psychiatric disorder focus on, and are distressed by, the somatic symptoms that accompany these disorders rather than the distressing thoughts or emotions characteristic of the disorder. All psychiatric disorders have symptoms that are "above the neck" (i.e., cognitive and emotional symptoms) and "below the neck" (i.e., somatic symptoms). Which symptom(s) a particular patient focuses on is influenced by many factors.

The most common diagnoses to present with physical symptoms are major depression (e.g., sleep disturbance, appetite disturbance, fatigue, pain) or an anxiety disorder. Panic disorder is the most likely anxiety disorder to present with somatic symptoms (e.g., palpitations, dyspnea, trembling, shaking, hot and cold flashes, lightheadedness).

A summary of major psychiatric disorders associated with somatization includes:
- major depression
- anxiety disorders:
  - panic disorder
  - generalized anxiety disorder
  - posttraumatic stress disorder
  - acute stress disorder
- substance abuse or dependence
- psychotic disorders:
  - schizophrenia
  - delusional disorder — somatic subtype.

Table 5.1 Important clinical characteristics of the somatoform disorder diagnoses

SOMATOFORM DIAGNOSIS	DIAGNOSTIC FEATURES
Somatization Disorder (SD)	Chronic, fluctuating disorder
	Onset before 30, typically in adolescence
	Symptoms may fluctuate over time but must include:
	Pain symptoms in four different sites (e.g., head, abdomen, back, joints, extremities, chest, rectum) *or associated with different functions* (e.g., menstruation, intercourse, urination)
	Two gastrointestinal symptoms (e.g., nausea, bloating, vomiting, diarrhea, food intolerance)
	One pseudoneurological symptom (e.g., impaired co-ordination or balance, paralysis or localized weakness, difficulty swallowing or lump in throat, aphonia, double vision, blindness, deafness, loss of sensation of touch or pain, seizures, or dissociative symptoms such as amnesia or loss of consciousness)
	One sexual symptom (e.g., irregular menses, menorrhagia, vomiting throughout pregnancy, erectile or ejaculatory dysfunction, sexual indifference)
Undifferentiated Somatoform Disorder	One or more unexplained physical complaints lasting for > 6 months

PREVALENCE	RISK FACTORS	COMMON COMORBIDITIES
Community: 0.2−2% of women, <0.2% of men Primary care: 1−5%	Genetic (SD in female and antisocial and substance abuse in male relatives) History of childhood victimization or parental neglect	High rates of psychiatric comorbidities Axis I − depression, panic disorder, substance abuse Axis II − borderline/narcissistic/antisocial (seen in psych settings) and avoidant/dependent/obsessive-compulsive (seen in primary care) Poor interpersonal relationships Multiple social problems Impaired psychosocial function
No studies of undifferentiated somatoform disorder but there are studies of subsyndromal somatization disorder where there is a community prevalence of 4−11%	Not well studied	Not well studied

Table 5.1 Somatoform disorder characteristics, continued

SOMATOFORM DIAGNOSIS	DIAGNOSTIC FEATURES
Hypochondriasis	Persistent fears of having a disease or belief that one has a disease based upon misinterpretation of one or more bodily symptoms despite medical reassurance Primary hypochondriasis appears to be a chronic condition. Secondary hypochondriasis can occur in the context of serious illness in patients or someone close to them, or during the course of another Axis I diagnosis (e.g., panic disorder, MDD).
Conversion Disorder	Typically abrupt, dramatic onset Symptoms involve voluntary motor or sensory functioning suggestive of a neurological or other medical illness ("pseudoneurological symptoms"). Symptoms are not intentionally produced. Psychological factors associated with onset or exacerbation.

PREVALENCE	RISK FACTORS	COMMON COMORBIDITIES
Community: 1–5% Ambulatory care: 4–6% Inpatient: 3–13% Most common onset is early adulthood.	Major life stress New onset medical disorder Other Axis I disorder with prominent physical symptoms (e.g., panic) Better prognosis with acute onset, brief duration, mild symptoms, presence of comorbid medical condition and lack of comorbid psychiatric condition	Bodily preoccupation is common—it may be with a particular bodily function (e.g., heartbeat), a trivial abnormal physical state (e.g., cough), a vague physical sensation, a particular organ or disease (e.g., cancer) High rates of Axis I comorbidities—GAD, panic disorder, MDD, dysthymic disorder, somatization disorder Exaggerated appraisal of risk of disease and belief that good health is a symptom-free state Interpersonal relationships deteriorate because of preoccupation with disease Iatrogenic complications because of unneeded medical investigations Impaired social and occupational functioning
Community: 0.3% Ambulatory care: 1–3% Hospitalized neurological or medical patients: 1–4.5% F > M 2:1 – 10:1	Severe social stressor(s) Antecedent illness serving as a model in patient or close contact Isolated, rural settings Developing countries Combat Industrial accidents	Poorly studied Frequent comorbid diagnoses include PTSD, depression, dissociative disorder, other somatoform disorders Long-standing conversion reactions may be associated with secondary physical sequelae (e.g., atrophy from disuse, decreased range of motion, etc.)

Table 5.1 Somatoform disorder characteristics, continued

SOMATOFORM DIAGNOSIS	DIAGNOSTIC FEATURES
Pain Disorder	Medically unexplained pain (pain in absence of medical disease or disproportionate to degree of pathology) that is the individual's chief complaint
	Psychological factors play significant role in onset, severity, exacerbation or maintenance of pain.
	Significant distress or impairment in social, occupational, or other important areas of functioning.
Body Dysmorphic Disorder	Preoccupation with an imagined defect in appearance or markedly excessive concern in the face of a slight physical anomaly. Intensity of preoccupation has been described as "torturing" or "tormenting."
	Frequent checking behaviours

PREVALENCE	RISK FACTORS	COMMON COMORBIDITIES
Very limited data	Very limited data	Little empirical data in discrete DSM-IV Pain Disorder patients but important to consider:
Estimates of 6 mo prevalence: 5%	Familial component with increased rates of depressive disorders, alcohol dependence and chronic pain in 1st degree biological relatives of Pain Disorder patients	Substance use disorders (esp. dependence or abuse of opioids or benzodiazepines)
Lifetime prevalence: 12%		Depression
F > M 2:1		Anxiety and anxiety disorders
	Depression is associated with subsequent development of chronic pain but hasn't been well documented re: Pain Disorder	Sleep disorders (obstructive sleep apnea, nocturnal myoclonus)
		Psychosocial dysfunction (social isolation, unemployment, marital and family difficulties)
Community: 0.7%	Poorly studied	Surgical correction is sought by approximately 75% and it may worsen BDD
Cosmetic surgery: 5–15%		Increased rate of Axis I comorbidities — MDD, social phobia, substance use disorders, OCD
Adolescent onset is most common.		
Differential focus of preoccupation by sex: women are more preoccupied with hips and weight and men with body build, genitals and thinning hair.		Increased rate of Axis II disorders with Cluster C avoidant most common
		Increased rate of suicide
		Profound psychosocial dysfunction

Undiagnosed physical disorder

Patients may be preoccupied by their bodies because there is something medically wrong with them.

Early presentations of a wide variety of diseases may be characterized by such non-specific symptoms as fatigue, decreased energy, sleep disturbance, abdominal discomfort, muscle aches, etc.

Consider functional somatic syndromes (see page 62).

Comorbidities

Patients with somatoform disorders have very high rates of comorbidity with other psychiatric diagnoses. Therefore, always screen for depression, panic disorder and generalized anxiety disorder. The likelihood of a given diagnosis in an individual patient varies considerably.

Factitious disorder and malingering

These are uncommon diagnoses. The patient who is somatizing experiences symptoms and is not involved in their production, in contrast to these two diagnoses where symptoms are intentionally produced for gain in malingering or for unconscious reasons (e.g., wish to occupy "sick role") in factitious disorder.

Rapid assessment

Unfortunately, rapid assessment is unrealistic in this group of patients. The only case where you may succeed in less than five minutes is with a well-known "thick chart" patient who comes in with a new, highly improbable symptom.

Plan to assess these patients over a minimum of several sessions. If possible, schedule an extended appointment for the assessment.

The basic assessment includes:
· a history of the presenting complaint
· a focused physical examination and relevant investigations.

When no organic basis is found for the symptom, do a "psychiatric review of systems" to rule out the common major psychiatric disorders presenting with prominent bodily complaints (see "Undiagnosed major psychiatric disorder," page 63). If a major psychiatric disorder is present, focus on treating that disorder with the hope that success will also address the reported physical symptoms.

If the patient does not have a common major psychiatric disorder, then consider the somatoform diagnoses summarized above (see "Somatoform disorders" on page 62 and Table 5.1 on page 64).

Patients who present with medically unexplained symptoms

Broadly speaking, there are two groups of patients who present with medically unexplained symptoms: patients you know, and patients who are new to your practice.

Patients you know

"THICK CHART" PATIENTS
The "thick chart" patient has had many medically unexplained symptoms with multiple past investigations and is well known to you.

Rule out an organic cause and a current major psychiatric disorder (see, "Undiagnosed major psychiatric disorder," page 63) and then review the clinical characteristics of somatoform disorders in Table 5.1 (page 64) and see where the patient most likely falls within the somatoform diagnoses.

PATIENTS PRESENTING WITH PERSISTENT, MEDICALLY UNEXPLAINED
SOMATIC COMPLAINT(S)

Check out recent psychosocial stressors without implying that the patient
is responsible for the stressor, or that the stressor is "causing" the symptom.
Questions likely to be of higher yield include: "Having symptoms like you
are describing is really difficult and makes it harder to put up with other
stress in your life. Are your symptoms making it difficult to cope with other
stresses right now?"

MUS may have developed in response to a high level of life stress, particularly a major medical illness in their partner, family or friends. Patients often
do not make what may seem like obvious connections. An example could
be a patient preoccupied with her bowel function over the last few months.
When asked about how her disturbed bowel function is impacting the
other stresses in her life, the patient replies that it is terribly difficult as she
is the executor for her uncle's estate. When asked what the uncle died of,
the patient responds, "colon cancer."

It is likely that these patients have a major psychiatric disorder (see
"Undiagnosed major psychiatric disorder," page 63), other than a somatoform
disorder, which accounts for their presentation. Do a careful review of
psychiatric symptomatology, especially depression and anxiety.

Patients who are new to your practice

· Do not assume that you will make a rapid assessment.
· Try to get at least some past medical records for more information.
· Start with ruling out organic pathology, then turn to ruling out a major
  psychiatric diagnosis. Finally, see if you can rule in a somatoform diagnosis.

Ruling out organic pathology

Ruling out organic pathology is important for several reasons:

1. You do not want to miss a treatable illness.

If patients have a somatoform diagnosis or MUS then you need to be comfortable managing them. This means that you need to be able to calmly reassure yourself that they do not have a treatable illness or illnesses when they present with multiple symptomatic complaints.

2. Patients need to know you are taking them seriously.

Patients who are somatizing typically need some initial investigations as evidence that you have taken them seriously and are not just brushing them off. Doing minimal but relevant investigations then opens the door for you to subsequently refuse other investigations unless medically indicated. While it may seem wasteful to do "medically unnecessary investigations," typically the "theatre" of doing so pays off many times over in that it helps to settle patients down and makes it more likely that they will follow your advice and not make unnecessary visits to the emergency room or walk-in clinics, or seek second opinions, and so forth. The health care dollars spent on these initial investigations are likely to save many more health care dollars in patients' pursuit of a health care professional who "takes them seriously." Draw the line at investigations that carry significant risk of harm.

What investigations do I order?

Start with baseline investigations indicated by the clinical complaint. Consider ordering second-line or more expensive investigations (e.g., CT scan) if there are clinical indications to do so or if you sense that the patient will not settle without having them done and there is a very low risk of harm associated with the procedure.

Be reasonable. Medical training focuses on the axiom "common things are common." Therefore, clinicians have been encouraged to think of horses when they hear hoofbeats. Nevertheless, our training also emphasizes the possibility of zebras. The combination of our own anxiety, our concerns about medico-legal risk, and our sincere desire to do the best for our patients makes it hard to know when to stop investigating unexplained somatic complaints. Usually, the best strategy is to do good baseline investigations and then to keep your ears open for a change in symptoms or further development of symptoms that sets off alarm bells and warrants further investigation.

Treatment options

General management approach with patients who are somatizing

- Reassure patients that you are not dismissing their symptoms and that you do not see the problem as "all in their head." Emphasize that you understand that they have distressing symptoms in their body and need relief and that you are trying to help them.
- Explain the results of their investigations (there is an art to doing this with these patients) and emphasize the importance of improving their functional status and quality of life in spite of their symptoms.
- Let them know that the investigations have reassured you that there is no evidence of a sinister condition or a biological abnormality requiring correction through a medication, specific treatment or surgery.
- Empathize with them that it is frustrating that at this point in the 21st century modern medicine cannot measure or image the symptoms they are experiencing.
- Emphasize that a negative finding on the tests is not equivalent to them "faking" or the symptom being "all in their head." Remind them that you take their symptoms seriously and that the distress they are experiencing is real and debilitating. The idea of their symptom(s) being a disorder of function rather than structure is often helpful to many patients.
- Reassure them that you will continue to follow them and work with them to decrease the level of their distress and improve the level of their functioning.
- Indicate that you will only do further investigations if they describe a symptom complex that raises a "red flag" or "sets off alarms" for you. These images are helpful as you move forward in terms of being able to say "no red flags or alarms" whenever you deny future pleas for more tests.

· Encourage forward movement. Emphasize that now that the investigations have demonstrated no sinister pathology, it is time to focus on managing their symptoms and building a satisfactory quality of life despite the symptoms.

ESTABLISH A TIME FOR REGULAR FOLLOW-UP
It is easier to work with patients who are somatizing when you do it on a schedule that works for them and for you.

Schedule follow-ups at the minimum interval between their current visits to your office using standing appointments. If they are arriving at your office once a week, make a weekly appointment at a time of day that works for you.

Regular follow-up removes from patients the sense that they need to present with a physical symptom or complaint in order to see a primary care provider. When you remove the need to present a symptom and you offer regular follow-up because "they have a lot of symptoms and are dealing with a lot" and you "want to help them," patients will gradually begin to focus less on their physical symptoms when they are with you.

At the regular follow-up appointments, allot a maximum of a couple of minutes for an update on physical symptoms and then insist that the conversation focus on activities that the patient has been involved in. Eventually, these sessions will come to feel more like social chats but they are in fact powerful reinforcers of the patient's increased functioning and a much more pleasant way for both of you to spend the time together that sustains them. Primary care providers new to this strategy often say, "But aren't I wasting the health care system's money by talking about _____ (e.g., cooking, children, sports, etc.)?" In fact, this strategy saves the health care system significant amounts of money since this approach will limit visits to emergency rooms, specialists, unnecessary investigations and increased drug costs.

Slowly increase the time between appointments as the patient "settles down." Take advantage of natural breaks, such as conference leaves or vacations, to increase the time between appointments. Be sure the patient has settled down before beginning to increase intervals or the situation will decompensate. For the most challenging of these patients, you will have to move very slowly and it may take a year or two before you can begin to space out appointments.

TREAT WHAT CAN BE TREATED
Treat major psychiatric disorders if they are present.

Patients with long-standing symptoms, a low level of functioning and significant deconditioning will benefit from a slow and graded physical reactivation. Get patients to keep a chart and record what they do each day. Walking is the best activity for most patients, as it is easy, has no cost and can be done without the need for equipment.

Establish a starting target for physical activity. There are two approaches to setting targets for physical activity:
· You can start with what your patients can do on their worst days and then have them do that every day.
· You can find out what they can comfortably do on an average day and then cut the time in half and have them begin by doing that every day.

For the most deconditioned, aim lower. For example, if patients can only walk to the bathroom on their worst days, then have them, as their reconditioning exercise, walk that distance every day for a week and then slowly increase their distance.

Increase their activity level in small increments. For example, increase their activity each week by a small amount (e.g., one or two minutes). If they are in fairly good physical condition, then they can progress more rapidly. The ultimate goal, for patients with no medical contraindications, is to get them into the cardiovascular training range where they will benefit from enhanced endorphin release and the positive benefits on mood (i.e., 30 minutes of exercise five days a week). This may take six months or more to achieve.

Symptomatic treatments (e.g., massage) may be helpful, but think carefully before you suggest them. Consider whether the treatment will be a bridge to increased function or if it may be construed as evidence of fragility. If patients are passive recipients of treatment, will this potentially undermine your attempts to have them assume more control over their lives?

EVALUATE AND TAILOR THEIR PHARMACOTHERAPY

These patients often have long lists of medications. Often it is because they have seen a variety of practitioners, each adding medications targeting various symptoms. Many patients with somatization disorder are on extensive "cocktails" of multiple opioids and benzodiazepines.

Make a list of all of the current standing medications and evaluate where there is overlap and assess the value of each medication, determining if it is benign or if it is associated with negative effects or side-effects. If possible, have patients bring in all of their medications and go through each agent with them to figure out how often they use it and under what conditions.

Make a list of all prn medications. Determine how often patients are using prn medications during the average "bad" and "not as bad/somewhat better" day. Check this against the rate at which they fill their prescription or ask them to monitor their use for a couple of weeks. Do their current prn medications make sense? Could their needs be better met with a standing medication?

Opioids and benzodiazepines need to be carefully evaluated. The crucial test with both of these medications is whether their use is associated with an improved level of function and an acceptable side-effect profile. Opioids are particularly problematic as, in addition to having well-known side-effects such as constipation and sedation, they may also be associated with hyperalgesia, rebound headaches and pain, and decreased testosterone. While a trial of opioids may be appropriate in the context of chronic non-malignant pain, their ongoing use needs to be supported by evidence of increased function. Many patients will require very slow, gradual tapers of these medications in order to function optimally.

Develop an optimal pharmacotherapy plan and then work over time to gradually get the patient there. It may take a year or more to rationalize the pharmacotherapy of many of these patients.

MANAGE YOUR OWN REACTION TO THE PATIENT

Most health care professionals find patients who are somatizing very challenging to work with. Each of us finds different aspects of their presentation more problematic: there can be minimal gratification as symptoms are not rapidly treated; irritation with their degree of disability in contrast to some of our patients with major medical illnesses who are coping in the face of considerable pain and morbidity; and difficult personality disorders that are over-represented in this patient group. Recognize that these patients can evoke negative feelings. The problem is not the negative feelings that we can handle professionally but rather the cases where we deny the negative feelings and then end up acting out on the patient. The following strategies can help to manage reactions to these challenging patients:

· Find something you can like about the patient or something intriguing about the patient.
· Take pleasure in small gains. Working with these patients is a slow process. We need to recognize when they have done something positive (e.g., the patient with somatization disorder who goes to a walk-in clinic in response to a new symptom rather than going to the emergency room).
· Remember that you should never be working harder at getting your patient better than the patient is working.
· Do something nice for yourself when you have had a particularly challenging encounter.
· Be realistic. Some patients are somatically preoccupied because it is the only alternative available for them in the context of their very challenging life circumstances. It may be impossible for them to shift their behaviour because it serves important functions in their lives.

Specific treatments for somatoform disorders

PSYCHOPHARMACOLOGY OF SOMATIZING DISORDERS
Psychopharmacology treatment may be directed to:
· treating a specific psychiatric disorder (e.g., depression or anxiety) that
  is either the primary cause of the somatic symptoms or occurs secondary
  to a somatoform disorder or functional somatic syndrome
· ameliorating specific target symptoms that may be addressed by psychopharmacology (e.g., sleep, fatigue)
· treating a somatoform disorder—while the evidence base continues to be
  sub-optimal, there is evidence that SSRIs may be helpful in patients with
  hypochondriasis, body dysmorphic disorder, somatization disorder and undifferentiated somatoform disorder; SNRIs may be helpful in pain disorder.

PSYCHOTHERAPY FOR PATIENTS WITH SOMATOFORM DISORDERS
Psychotherapeutic approaches to somatoform disorders include a wide
variety of psychotherapeutic models and techniques. Unfortunately, it is
difficult to find therapists skilled or interested in using these therapies with
patients with somatoform disorders. The evidence base for psychotherapeutic treatment of somatoform disorders remains limited. In deciding
about therapy, it is helpful to consider the following points:
· Cognitive-behavioural therapy (CBT) is the best-studied psychotherapy
  for this group of patients. It is helpful in the management of hypochondriasis
  and pain disorder with a significant psychological component. CBT has
  documented value in the care of patients with a variety of functional
  somatic syndromes. Unfortunately, finding practitioners skilled in these
  modalities is often a struggle. If the patient is receiving disability benefits,
  an advocacy letter to his or her disability insurer may result in funding for
  a course of CBT with an appropriately trained psychologist.
· Could the patient benefit from general supportive therapy? This is often
  useful, especially when patients are experiencing high levels of life stress and
  have poor social supports. If you are willing and able to make time in your
  practice to see them, you may wish to provide the support. The key strategy
  is to make follow-up consistent and predictable. Alternatively, you may serve
  them best by monitoring the medical aspects of the situation and referring

them to a GP psychotherapist, the local mental health clinic or a family service association for support.

- Insight-oriented psychotherapies are helpful in a select group of these patients who show an ability to form a therapeutic relationship and display a degree of psychological mindedness.
- Family or marital therapy may be of benefit when these issues form a prominent part of the individual's presentation.
- Relaxation therapies may be of value in decreasing the physiological consequences of stress (e.g., muscle tension) and may thus decrease symptom burden.
- Mindfulness-based stress reduction may be helpful in terms of assisting patients to manage their stress better and to lead their lives despite their symptoms.
- Support groups, especially those without professional facilitation, cannot be wholly recommended, specifically because some are very helpful while others are unhelpful. Support groups that focus on how sick and dysfunctional everyone is are particularly unhelpful as they emphasize passivity and undermine your goal of increasing the patient's functional status. Ask patients about the perspective of the support groups they attend and start to get an idea about which groups in your community are likely to be helpful.

Helping the patient's family

Patients' families often struggle given the significant degree to which symptoms dominate the lives of patients who somatize and render them dysfunctional.

- Encourage family members to have their own support if needed.
- Assess whether marital or family therapy is needed.
- Explain that how we respond to another's behaviour can make that behaviour either more or less likely in the future. We can inadvertently reinforce dysfunction and passivity when we provide attention or support for behaviours of inactivity and disability. Similarly, we can reinforce positive behaviours by providing attention and praise to those behaviours.

When to refer to a psychiatrist

Typically, patients with somatoform disorders cannot readily find treatment within psychiatry because most psychiatrists have little training in assessing or managing these disorders. Further, most psychiatrists are not interested in these patients as they find them frustrating to work with because these patients focus on physical symptoms and their treatment is usually slow.

If you are lucky enough to have access to a psychiatrist, he or she may be helpful in terms of:

· assessing suicidal risk, which develops in some patients given the frequently bleak nature of their lives with unremitting physical symptomatology and the high burden of other psychiatric comorbidity

· giving advice about the management of treatment-resistant depression or anxiety that may be either the primary issue or a secondary comorbidity with a somatoform disorder

· confirming a diagnosis. Be forewarned though that many psychiatrists are uncomfortable with evaluating physical symptoms and medical issues and recommend more medical investigations for that reason. Sometimes, more investigations are appropriate and a fresh set of eyes and ears may find some evidence of organicity that needs to be pursued. At other times, more investigations are a balm for the psychiatrist's anxiety at his or her distance from the day-to-day evaluation of physical symptomatology and the psychiatrist may disrupt your attempts to limit investigations.

Preparing the patient for a psychiatric consultation

Preparing patients for a psychiatric consultation is important, given the lingering stigma and misperceptions that continue to exist about psychiatry.

Indicate that you want to give the best care possible to your patients, that their symptoms are important, that their suffering is real and that your care will be improved and you will feel better if the patient sees a colleague with expertise in _____ (e.g., assessing risk of suicide, the use of medications that were initially developed for the treatment of anxiety and depression but are often quite effective in managing symptoms that the patient is experiencing such as fatigue and sleep problems, improving quality of life in people with significant physical symptoms that interfere with their life, etc.).

Anticipate for patients that their referral to psychiatry may be experienced negatively—either in the moment, or when they get home and have a chance to think about it as evidence that you really think it is "all in their head" or that you are trying to "dump them." If there is a negative reaction, ask patients to remind themselves that the referral is a sign of your caring for them and wanting the best for them and that you are committed to their ongoing management.

If the psychiatrist is someone who sees a number of medically ill patients, add that to your "sell" (e.g., "Dr. X has been helpful to me and my patients with a whole range of physical problems, including problems such as you have, and has also helped to improve the quality of life of patients of mine with cancer and heart disease"). This will help patients to not immediately dismiss the psychiatrist as someone who "won't know anything" about physical symptoms.

Community and online resources
Unfortunately, there are no specific community resources directed toward these patients in most communities.

There are few clinically helpful online resources.
· American Academy of Family Physicians, Somatoform Disorders fact sheet for patients: http://familydoctor.org/online/famdocen/home/common/pain/disorders/162.html

References

Abbey, S.E. (2005). Somatization and somatotoform disorders. In J.L. Levenson (Ed.), *The American Psychiatric Publishing Textbook Of Psychosomatic Medicine* (pp. 271–296). Arlington, VA: American Psychiatric Publishing.

Abbey, S.E. (2010). Assessment of patients with somatization. In D.S. Goldbloom (Ed.), *Psychiatric Clinical Skills* (Rev. 1st ed.; pp. 187–203). Toronto: Centre for Addiction and Mental Health.

American Psychiatric Association. (2000). *Diagnostic and Statistical Manual of Mental Disorders* (4th ed., text rev.). Washington DC: Author.

Calabrese, L. & Stern, T.A. (2004). The patient with multiple medical complaints. In T.A. Stern, J.B. Herman & P.L. Slavin (Eds.), *Massachusetts General Hospital Guide to Primary Care Psychiatry* (page 269–278). New York: McGraw-Hill Medical Publishing Division.

Looper, K.J. & Kirmayer, L.J. (2002). Behavioral medicine approaches to somatoform disorders. *Journal of Consulting and Clinical Psychology, 70*, 810–827.

Sumathipala, A. (2007). What is the evidence for the efficacy of treatments for somatoform disorders? A critical review of previous intervention studies. *Psychosomatic Medicine, 69* (9), 889–900.

6

The patient with a substance use problem

AGNES KWASNICKA AND PETER SELBY

Brief overview of differential diagnosis

Patients rarely present seeking help for substance use disorders. They are more likely to present with a medical, psychological or social condition caused by their substance use. Thus substance use should be part of the differential diagnosis for a variety of medical and psychiatric disorders. Substance use does not equal addiction or a substance-related disorder. However, it is necessary to differentiate these conditions because the management and prognosis are different.

Definitions

PROBLEM DRINKING

Problem drinking is not a DSM-IV diagnosis but is commonly used to refer to alcohol consumption that is greater than low-risk drinking guidelines (see Table 6.1). In problem drinking there are potential social, physical or psychological consequences, but DSM criteria for Abuse or Dependence are not met.

Note that there are significant international variations in standard drink size and in the definition of risk.

Table 6.1 Low-risk drinking guidelines

MEN	WOMEN
maximum 15 standard drinks (SD) per week, 0–3 SD per day.	maximum of 10 SD per week, 0–2 SD per day.

1 SD = 43 mL (1.5 oz.) 40% strength spirits; 142 mL (5 oz.) 12.5% strength table wine; 341 mL (12 oz.) 5% strength beer.

(Butt et al., 2010)

Note: there are no low-risk guidelines for other substances.

DSM-IV-TR Criteria for Substance Abuse

A. A maladaptive pattern of substance use leading to clinically significant impairment or distress, as manifested by one (or more) of the following, occurring within a 12-month period:

   (1) recurrent substance use resulting in a failure to fulfill major role obligations at work, school, or home (e.g., repeated absences or poor work performance related to substance use; substance-related absences, suspensions, or expulsions from school; neglect of children or household)

   (2) recurrent substance use in situations in which it is physically hazardous (e.g., driving an automobile or operating a machine when impaired by substance use)

   (3) recurrent substance-related legal problems (e.g., arrests for substance-related disorderly conduct)

   (4) continued substance use despite having persistent or recurrent social or interpersonal problems caused or exacerbated by the effects of the substance (e.g., arguments with a spouse about the consequences of intoxication, physical fights)

B. The symptoms have never met the criteria for Substance Dependence for this class of substance.

Reprinted with permission from the *Diagnostic and Statistical Manual of Mental Disorders, Fourth Edition, Text Revision* (Copyright 2000). American Psychiatric Association.

Abbreviated criteria for substance abuse can be recalled by using the "SLOP" mnemonic (Selby & Handford, 2010):
· use despite harm (**S**ocial consequences)
· **L**egal problems
· failure to fulfill major roles (**O**bligations)
· recurrent use in **P**hysically hazardous situations.

DSM-IV-TR Criteria for Substance Dependence

A maladaptive pattern of substance use, leading to clinically significant impairment or distress, as manifested by three (or more) of the following, occurring at any time in the same 12-month period:

(1) tolerance, as defined by either of the following:

  (a) a need for markedly increased amounts of the substance to achieve intox-ication or the desired effect

  (b) markedly diminished effect with continued use of the same amount of the substance

(2) withdrawal, as manifested by either of the following:

  (a) the characteristic withdrawal syndrome for the substance

  (b) the same (or a closely related) substance is taken to relieve or avoid withdrawal symptoms

(3) the substance is often taken in larger amounts or over a longer period than was intended

(4) there is a persistent desire or unsuccessful efforts to cut down or control substance use

(5) a great deal of time is spent in activities necessary to obtain the substance (e.g., visiting multiple doctors or driving long distances), use the substance (e.g., chain-smoking), or recover from its effects

(6) important social, occupational, or recreational activities are given up or reduced because of substance use

(7) the substance use is continued despite knowledge of having a persistent or recurrent physical or psychological problem that is likely to have been caused or exacerbated by the substance (e.g., current cocaine use despite recognition of cocaine-induced depression, or continued drinking despite recognition that an ulcer was made worse by alcohol consumption)

Reprinted with permission from the *Diagnostic and Statistical Manual of Mental Disorders*, Fourth Edition, Text Revision (Copyright 2000). American Psychiatric Association.

The abbreviated criteria for dependence can be recalled by using the WET TICK mnemonic (Selby & Handford, 2010):
· **W**ithdrawal
· **E**xcessive use (time and/or quantity)
· **T**olerance
· a great deal of **T**ime spent acquiring, using or recovering from the substance
· **I**nterference with roles
· inability to **C**ut down
· continued use despite **K**nowledge of harm.

CONCURRENT DISORDER
A concurrent disorder is defined as a concurrent psychiatric and substance use disorder. In the present context, the term "concurrent disorder" is distinct from "dual diagnosis," which refers to the presence of both a psychiatric disorder and a developmental delay.

INTOXICATION AND WITHDRAWAL
Intoxication and withdrawal are characterized by the following:
· The development of a reversible substance-specific syndrome due to recent ingestion of or exposure to a substance (*intoxication*) or cessation of or reduction in use of a substance (*withdrawal*).
· The substance-specific syndrome causes either of the following:
  - **Intoxication**: clinically significant maladaptive behavioural or psychological changes that are due to the *effect of the substance* on the central nervous system (e.g., belligerence, mood lability, cognitive impairment, impaired

judgment, impaired social or occupational functioning) and develop
during or shortly after use of the substance.
- **Withdrawal**: clinically significant distress or impairment in social,
  occupational or other important areas of functioning *due to the absence*
  of the drug.
· The symptoms are *not* due to a general *medical* condition and are not
  better accounted for by another *mental* disorder.

TOLERANCE
Tolerance is characterized by the need for greatly increased amounts of
the substance to achieve intoxication (or the desired effect) or a markedly
diminished effect with continued use of the same amount of the substance.

POLYSUBSTANCE DEPENDENCE
Polysubstance dependence is diagnosed when a person uses three or more
substances (with the exception of caffeine and tobacco) and meets criteria
for dependence. No single substance accounts for the problems experienced
by the patient.

How to make the diagnosis in less than five minutes (rapid assessment)

Key questions
IS THE PATIENT INTOXICATED (MILD TO SEVERE) OR IN WITHDRAWAL?
Intoxication, the immediate influence of a drug, is specific to a particular
drug or class of drug while withdrawal is a distinct syndrome characteristic
of the discontinuation of a substance.

As a general rule, intoxication with stimulants (e.g., cocaine, metham-
phetamine) leads to increased arousal while withdrawal is associated
with somnolence. The opposite is true with depressant drugs (e.g.,
opioids, benzodiazepines).

IS SUBSTANCE USE INVOLVED?

When a patient presents with any psychiatric condition, screening for substance use is necessary. In addition, the following physical conditions are red flags for possible substance use.

General:
· fatigue
· weight loss
· hypertension
· frequent trauma
· odour of alcohol on breath

GI:
· hepatitis
· gastritis
· pancreatitis

Renal:
· frequency
· hematuria
· shrunken bladder

Neurological:
· seizures
· tremors

Respiratory:
· chronic cough

Infections:
· HIV
· HCV
· HBV

· sexually transmitted infections (STIs)
· infective endocarditis
· signs of injection drug use (e.g., "track marks")

Obstetric:
· IUGR
· recurrent pregnancy loss

Social and family:
· divorce
· child protection agency involvement
· spousal abuse

Occupational, legal and/or economic:
· job loss
· impaired driving
· arrest
· sudden loss of money
· poor school performance

Screening for alcohol and drug problems in all patients

Ask all patients over nine years of age about alcohol, tobacco, prescription (e.g., benzodiazepines, opioids), over-the-counter (e.g., dimenhydrinate, acetaminophen with codeine) and street drug use (e.g., cocaine, cannabis, and heroin).

Screening questionnaires can help to quickly identify a substance use problem or determine the level of dependence. Once a substance use disorder is identified or suspected, additional questions should be used to learn more about the degree of use, consequences the patient may have experienced and the patient's readiness to engage in treatment.

Table 6.2 The CAGE questionnaire adapted to include drugs (CAGE-AID)

1. Have you felt you ought to **C**ut down on your drinking or drug use?

2. Have people **A**nnoyed you by criticizing your drinking or drug use?

3. Have you felt bad or **G**uilty about your drinking or drug use?

4. Have you ever had a drink or used drugs first thing in the morning to steady your nerves or to get rid of a hangover (**E**ye-opener)?

Score: __ /4

2/4 or greater = positive CAGE, further evaluation is indicated.

Reprinted with permission from the *Wisconsin Medical Journal*. Brown, R.L. and Rounds, L.A. Conjoint screening questionnaires for alcohol and other drug abuse. *Wisconsin Medical Journal* 94:135–140, 1995.

Implementing effective screening strategies

Patients often have difficultly disclosing and quantifying their use. Inquiring about *how much* they use rather than *if* they use gives them permission to be more honest.

Some other strategies to overcome the shame, fear or reluctance to disclose patients may feel include:

Preparing the patient for the question

"To better understand your condition I am going to ask you questions about your use of alcohol, tobacco and other drugs. Is that okay with you?"

Normalizing substance use

"Some people who suffer from anxiety self-medicate with alcohol to help them cope. Does this describe your situation?"

Overestimating the amount
"How many beers can you drink before you feel high? Is it closer to 24 or 12?"

Abuse of prescription medications: Red flags
In cases of suspected abuse of prescription medications, it is helpful to be alert to indicators of potentially problematic use. Abuse of prescribed medications may be encountered, for example, when treating a patient with an anxiety disorder with benzodiazepines or when treating a patient with chronic pain with opioids.

Features suggestive of problematic prescription drug use include:
· running out of medications early, presenting as:
  - multiple dose escalations with no evidence of benefit
  - multiple episodes of prescription "loss"
  - "borrowing" from family and friends
  - seeking prescriptions from multiple sources
· deterioration in functioning
· refusal to consider other treatment options despite lack of benefit.

What is the severity of the disorder?
The severity of the disorder is judged by its effects on various domains of the person's life. These include:
· impacts on physical health
· mental health and social functioning
· financial impacts
· failures in occupational/educational and/or other role responsibilities.

In the DSM-IV-TR, the less severe form is Substance Abuse while the more severe form is Substance Dependence.

Once a patient has met criteria for Dependence they can never meet criteria for Abuse again. A return to substance use after abstinence is considered a relapse to Dependence.

INTOXICATION

The most severe form of intoxication is considered an overdose and is a medical emergency. There is u sually respiratory compromise, disorientation and a reduced level of consciousness. Overdose with stimulants is associated with psychosis, seizures and cardiac arrhythmias.

WITHDRAWAL

Severe withdrawal, especially from alcohol, is associated with delirium (delirium tremens) and is characterized by illusions not visual hallucinations (i.e., misinterpreting environmental stimuli, for example, by mistaking a rope for a snake). It may be complicated by seizures as well. Opioid withdrawal, when severe, is characterized by autonomic symptoms including diarrhea, vomiting, sweating and pilo-erection. Seizures or delirium are not part of the opioid withdrawal syndrome.

TOBACCO

For tobacco use, the number of cigarettes smoked per day and how quickly someone smokes after waking is a guide to the level of dependence. People who smoke 10 or more cigarettes per day and have their first cigarette within five minutes of waking are considered severely dependent.

Can I verify the history?

Substance use disorders are best diagnosed by a thorough interview corroborated by a third party where possible and a focused physical examination. Often, the diagnosis is made prospectively and requires repeated visits. The following can be used to support a diagnosis or exclude potential contributors to a patient's presentation.

Direct measures

URINE DRUG SCREENING (UDS)

Urine is an ideal matrix to test for drugs of abuse. Patient consent is necessary except in emergencies. The more specific the request, the more likely the drug will be detected by the laboratory (e.g., oxycodone rather than opioid). Presence or absence of drug in UDS does not rule in or out a diagnosis of a substance use disorder (i.e., abuse or dependence). Depending on the time lapsed since last use, laboratory method, urine concentration, contamination and cut-off thresholds, the drug may not be detected. Therefore, UDS results *must* be interpreted in light of the clinical presentation.

BREATHALYSER
Breathalysers are rarely used in primary care. They are used more commonly in ER and law enforcement settings. However, this can be a useful tool if office-based withdrawal management is planned.
· Breathalysers detect blood alcohol concentration (BAC) in mg% (mg/100mL).
· Alveolar concentration of alcohol correlates closely to blood alcohol level.
· 1 mg% = 0.2175 mmol/L or 4.6 mg% =1 mmol/L.
· It is a criminal offence in Canada to drive having a BAC of ≥ 80 mg%.
· 160 mg% (equivalent to 34 mmol/L) is associated with clinically obvious intoxication in a non-tolerant individual.

BAC can vary substantially with consumption of the same amount of alcohol depending on a person's age, race, gender, weight, genetic predisposition or metabolic rate. More importantly, because of differing alcohol tolerance among individuals, it does not establish the patient's level of intoxication. Someone with significantly high tolerance can experience withdrawal symptoms even at BAC that would cause relatively intolerant individuals to exhibit sign of intoxication.

PHYSICAL SIGNS
The signs of substance use and substance use disorders are protean and depend on the type and number of drug(s) used, time since use and co-occurring psychiatric and physical disorders.

In acute care settings, it is important to assess vital signs, level of consciousness and level of orientation. The physical exam should focus on stigmata of drug use (e.g., "track marks"), usually related to the route of admission. Clinicians should correlate the observed level of impairment with the apparent level of consumption. They should have a high index of suspicion that other factors (i.e., subdural hematoma), might better account for or contribute to the clinical picture.

Pinpoint pupils with altered levels of consciousness and hypoventilation can indicate the use of opioids, while goosebumps, lacrimation, yawning and chills indicate opioid withdrawal. Ataxia and dysarthria are associated with alcohol intoxication while tremors and sweats are associated with alcohol withdrawal. Intoxication with stimulants is associated with restlessness, anorexia, paranoia and delusions. Withdrawal is associated with somnolence and increased hunger.

The physical examination is helpful but not diagnostic of a substance use disorder but more indicative of the effects of substance use.

Indirect measures

ALCOHOL
MCV and GGT
Gamma glutamyl transferase (GGT) and mean cell volume (MCV) both have low sensitivity for detecting alcohol problems; thus, a normal value should not be used as evidence to rule out an alcohol problem. Nonetheless, these are useful measures to confirm clinical suspicion and to monitor treatment response. MCV normalizes after three months and GGT normalizes after four weeks.

TOBACCO
Breath carbon monoxide monitor
The carbon monoxide (CO) found in cigarette smoke is absorbed via the lungs of people who smoke. CO competes with oxygen for hemoglobin, binding and displacing it, resulting in less oxygen delivery to tissue and vital organs. A convenient office detector measures breath CO in parts per million as an indirect measure of serum carboxyhemoglobin level (COHb). It can be used in smoking cessation counselling as a motivator to illustrate

to the patient the impact of their cessation efforts, or to verify self-reported smoking quantity. Other sources of CO (e.g., automobile exhaust) and time from last cigarette will also affect readings. CO levels of greater than 3ppm are found in people who smoke.

What is the relationship between substance use and presentation?

CONSEQUENCES OF SUBSTANCE USE
In addition to quantifying the amount, frequency, route and duration of use, it is important to explore the consequences of substance use in the person's life. To make the diagnosis, cautiously explore the link between substance use and the presenting complaint.

CONCURRENT DISORDERS
When patients who are abusing substances present with psychiatric symptoms, it may not be possible in the acute situation to differentiate between a substance-induced psychiatric disorder and a concurrent disorder.

Exploring the temporal relationship between substance use and the psychiatric symptoms may be helpful, but not always fruitful. Sometimes the relationship between substance use and the psychiatric symptoms can only be determined retrospectively, after substance use is significantly reduced or after weeks of abstinence. The inability to determine if the mental illness is distinct from the substance use disorder does not preclude treating the mental health issues concurrently with the substance use disorder.

What is the motivation for change? What is stage of change?

Counselling a patient who is using substances about treatment options is not a good use of a primary care provider's time if the patient is not yet ready to change. Every attempt should be made to match the intervention to the patient's stage of change (see Table 6.3 on page 98).

Table 6.3 Matching interventions to the stage of change

STAGE OF CHANGE	INDICATOR OF THE STAGE	APPROPRIATE INTERVENTION FOR THE STAGE	SAMPLE QUESTIONS
Pre-contemplation	May be defensive or uninterested in change May feel hopeless about change	Develop trusting relationship Raise doubt Increase perception of risk	*"How do you feel about your use of …?"* *"What does using … do for you?"*
Contemplation	Ambivalent Aware of pros and cons but has not acted	Acknowledge ambivalence and try to tip the balance Evoke reasons for change Strengthen self-efficacy	*"What are some of the good things about using …?"* *"What are some of the not-so-good things about using …?"*
Preparation	Committed to change Starting to make plans	Help plan: identify strengths, barriers, vulnerabilities Provide information and treatment choices	*"What was difficult last time you tried quitting?"* *"What are other changes you've successfully made?"*
Action	Implementing plans and making genuine efforts to change	Help patient take steps toward change Focus on the positive Help plan for high-risk situations	*"How do you feel about the changes you've made so far?"* *"What would you do in a triggering situation?"*

| Maintenance | Has had a period of time not using and is trying not to relapse | Help patient identify strategies to prevent relapse | *"What are changes you've made in your life to help you continue not using?"* |
| Relapse | Stopped for a period of time, but is now using the substance again | Help minimize degree and duration of relapse

Assist patient in identifying reasons for relapse | *"What was happening in your life when you started using again?"* |

ASSESS IMPORTANCE
Ask the patient:
"Given everything else going on in your life right now, how important is it for you to stop drinking/smoking/using drugs? Use a 10-point scale where 1 is 'not at all important' and 10 is 'the most important thing in life.' "

ASSESS CONFIDENCE
Ask the patient:
"How confident are you that you will be successful in your attempt to quit/cut down, on a scale of 1 to 10?"

ASSESS READINESS
Finally, ask the patient:
"How ready are you, on a scale of 1 to 10, to take steps toward changing your behaviour?"

Patients who rate high importance, confidence and readiness are more likely to succeed in their efforts to change their substance use. Assessing these variables allows the clinician to target motivational interventions to those that are rated low. Exploring risks and rewards of substance use can create discrepancy and increase readiness to change.

Follow any of these questions with: *"What would increase your importance/confidence/readiness just a little bit, from 6 to 7 for example?"* This strategy can be used to identify potential targets for intervention.

How to reasonably rule out underlying organic pathology

When a patient presents with psychiatric symptoms, it is critical to rule out an organic condition that may mimic a mental illness. In the case of substance use, the substance itself is often the organic cause for the presentation. To differentiate symptoms that can be attributed to organic pathology, or substance use, or both, it may be necessary to observe the patient. For instance:

- A patient who is dependent on alcohol may appear to be acutely intoxicated when in fact the patient has a subdural hematoma. In these circumstances, the BAC is much lower than expected.
- A patient with visual hallucinations may have intra-cerebral pathology, psychotic illness or alcohol withdrawal.
- A patient who uses cocaine and is experiencing weight loss may have underlying cancer.

Other questions to consider when differentiating organic versus psychiatric etiology

- Can a drug cause the signs and symptoms this patient is exhibiting?
- Can the signs and symptoms be attributed to withdrawal from a substance?
- Does the history of the amount consumed fit with the clinical presentation?

Treatment

Acute setting

Appropriate treatment of intoxication and withdrawal can be an ideal way to engage the patient in discussion about rehabilitation. Poorly treated withdrawal can perpetuate addiction as patients know how to relieve uncomfortable symptoms by resuming use of their drug of choice.

WITHDRAWAL MANAGEMENT (WM)

Determine if the patient requires medically supervised withdrawal management.

- Alcohol and benzodiazepine withdrawal generally require medical treatment due to risk of seizure.
- Patients with multiple medical problems are best monitored in a medical setting.
- Patients who are pregnant or those at risk of suicide should not be treated in an outpatient setting.
- Most other patients can be treated at a non-medical withdrawal management centre.

Is office-based or home withdrawal management appropriate?

- Management of uncomplicated alcohol or opioid withdrawal can often be done in a physician's office (see page 103).
- Home withdrawal management should only be attempted if the patient has stable housing, has a supportive family member or friend and is able to follow up in subsequent days.
- A degree of trust and background knowledge of the patient is strongly recommended.

Have a follow-up plan for rehabilitation before or early in withdrawal management. On its own, managed withdrawal is ineffective in maintaining long-term remission (see next section).

Rehabilitation

Early engagement of the patient is important for achieving treatment retention. Early engagement is associated with improved outcomes since active treatment is required to assist the patient maintain a drug-free life. This is usually a life-long commitment with increased intensity in the first year with gradual tapering of involvement as the person is able to maintain his or her goal. In harm reduction paradigms, the goal is to improve functioning in all domains without *requiring* complete abstinence from drug use.

Treatment options and setting

Tailoring treatment to the patient's lifestyle and other responsibilities has a greater chance of success and patient retention. Treatment programs are often organized by substance of use or other demographic factors (e.g., women-only groups, patients with concurrent psychiatric illness, etc.).

Outpatient day or evening programs
· These programs are often affiliated with hospitals or social service agencies.

Residential programs
· Duration varies from short (21 day) to long-term (up to six months) programs.
· Residential programs often provide ongoing group or individual support after completion of program.

Mutual aid groups
· Twelve-step-based mutual aid groups may have a spiritual or religious focus, or they may be secular.

Psychotherapy and counselling

Basic counselling can be provided even in a busy family practice. Perhaps the most important elements of counselling are a trusting relationship with the patient and an open-minded approach. The primary care provider's relationship with the patient and knowledge of the patient's background is invaluable.

Individual
· Individual counselling can be with a psychiatrist, GP psychotherapist, family physician, psychologist, social worker or other trained therapist.

Group
· Groups provide social support, acceptance, mentoring and practical advice.
· Groups may be inappropriate for some patients (e.g., severe social phobia, low functioning psychotic illness).

Motivational interviewing
· This directive, patient-centred counselling style elicits behavioural change by helping individuals explore and resolve ambivalence.
· Using the concept of the stages of change, this technique is oriented toward reaching goals and moving through the stages (i.e., from Pre-contemplation to Action to Maintenance).

Other counselling techniques
· Settings and approaches vary widely, thus knowledge of local community resources is advantageous.

Pharmacotherapy

Alcohol
ALCOHOL DEPENDENCE
Pharmacotherapy for alcohol dependence can easily be prescribed by the primary care physician (see Table 6.4). It should always be paired with at least brief counselling or, if available, a structured treatment program.

ACUTE WITHDRAWAL
The severity of withdrawal varies depending on the individual. For this reason, the amount of medication used to treat a person in acute withdrawal from alcohol should be flexible. The evidence suggests that all benzodiazepines are equally efficacious. However, diazepam is commonly used because of its long half-life (40 hours) that results in a pharmacokinetic self-taper after loading, translating into a smoother withdrawal and fewer rebound symptoms.

Table 6.4 Pharmacotherapy for alcohol dependence*

MEDICATION FEATURES	CONTRA-INDICATIONS	DOSE	MONITORING	DURATION OF THERAPY
Naltrexone (Revia)				
Opioid receptor antagonist

Decreases craving for alcohol and minimizes relapse if it occurs | Acute hepatitis or liver failure, caution in cirrhosis

Opoid dependence | 25 mg × 3d

then 50 mg qd

may increase to max 150 mg qd | At high doses can cause reversible elevations in transaminases

Frequency of monitoring is determined by baseline levels** | 3–6 months*** |
| **Acamprosate (Campral)** | | | | |
| Glutamate receptor modulator

Reduces symptoms of post-acute withdrawal (e.g., insomnia, anxiety and restlessness) | Severe renal impairment | 666 mg tid | No laboratory monitoring needed

Monitor for diarrhea (a common adverse effect) | Up to 1 year

Re-evaluate q3m |

Disulfiram (Antabuse)

If alcohol is con-sumed, causes toxic build-up of acetaldehyde by binding to acetaldehyde dehydrogenase	Unstable angina, recent MI	125–250 mg hs	Transaminases at baseline, 2 weeks then monthly × 3m	3–6 months***
	Schizophrenia and other psy-chotic illness			
Potentially fatal reaction	Pregnancy			
	Severe cir-rhosis			
	Precautions with many diseases			

*Combination therapy no more effective than monotherapy.

** If < 1.5 × normal repeat monthly × three months, less frequently thereafter; if 1.5–3 × normal repeat in two weeks; if > 3 × normal or elevated bilirubin withhold medication and repeat in two weeks.

*** Treatment can be continued after six months if no adverse effects.

Symptoms are assessed using the Clinical Institute Withdrawal Assessment for Alcohol (CIWA-Ar) (Sullivan et al., 1989). For patients who have a CIWA-Ar score of 10 or more or who are experiencing disorientation and/or hallucinosis, benzodiazepines should be used. A typical CIWA-Ar protocol is to give 20 mg po every hour until symptoms ameliorate. Assessment of the patient should occur prior to each dose. Diazepam loading via symptoms scores is safe and can be done as an outpatient. Suggest to the patient that he or she should stop drinking alcohol the evening before and come to the physician's office in the morning. Up to 60 mg (three doses) can be given over three hours. If the patient needs further benzodiazepines, the patient should be considered for inpatient management. Other indications for admission include delirium tremens, fever over 38 degrees Celsius, medical illness needing treatment, Wernicke's encephalopathy, and other drug dependency such as barbiturates and benzodiazepines. Generally, if there is a history of withdrawal seizures, 20 mg of diazepam should be given every hour for three consecutive doses. For those with severe asthma, respiratory failure, or liver disease, a shorter acting benzodiazepine (oxazepam or lorazepam) is recommended.

Opioids

Methadone
· In Canada, exemption from the *Controlled Drugs and Substances Act* (1996) is needed to prescribe methadone. Local provincial regulators set guidelines and regulations.
· Methadone is well supported by large cohort studies for treatment of opioid dependence.
· Treatment is often long-term (months to years).
· Methadone has a narrow therapeutic window with risk of overdose especially in non-tolerant individuals.

Buprenorphine
· Buprenorphine, an opioid receptor partial agonist, is available in Canada as buprenorphine/naloxone combination.
· While training and education are strongly encouraged before prescribing buprenorphine, physicians are not required to seek an exemption from Health Canada as they do if they decide to prescribe methadone.
· Compared with methadone:
  - less likely to cause an overdose due to the so-called "ceiling effect"
  - more rapid titration possible
  - milder withdrawal during tapering.

Tobacco
Pharmacotherapy doubles the chances of quitting per given quit attempt. Table 6.5 shows first-line treatments as per U.S. guidelines and Cochrane reviews giving the level of evidence and official indication for the treatment of tobacco dependence.

Table 6.5 Pharmacotherapy for smoking cessation

PHARMACO-THERAPY	DOSE	DURATION	EFFICACY VS. PLACEBO (OR [95% CI])*	MAJOR SIDE-EFFECTS
Nicotine replacement				
Patch	Available in 7, 14 and 21 mg Dose determined by cigarettes per day (CPD); some will need >1 patch If > 14 CPD use 21 mg	6 weeks on dose that controls withdrawal symptoms, then taper slowly (approx. q2wks)	1.77 [1.66–1.88] 1.81 [1.63–2.02] *at 6–12 months follow-up*	Skin irritation Nightmares
Gum	Available in 2 or 4 mg 1 piece q1–2h prn to max 24/d	As above, best used in conjunction with patch for breakthrough cravings	1.66 [1.52–1.81] *at 6–12 months follow-up*	GI side-effects if nicotine is swallowed
Inhaler	Cartridge contains 10 mg but delivers 4 mg nicotine q1–2h prn		2.14 [1.44–3.18] *at 6–12 months follow-up*	Mouth and throat irritation

Table 6.5 Pharmacotherapy, continued

PHARMACO-THERAPY	DOSE	DURATION	EFFICACY VS. PLACEBO (OR [95% CI])*	MAJOR SIDE-EFFECTS
Bupropion (Zyban)	To be started 1 week before quit day 150 mg qd day 1–3 150 mg bid thereafter (may continue qd if side-effects at bid dose)	Up to 12 weeks	1.94 [1.72–2.19] 1.07 [0.87–1.32]	Insomnia, headache, jitteriness Seizure (rare)
Varenicline (Champix)	Start 1 week before quit day 0.5 mg qd × 3d, then bid × 4d, 1 mg bid thereafter	12 weeks +/- additional 12 weeks if effective	2.82 [2.06–3.86]	Nausea, insomnia, headache, flatulence. May be associated with neuro-psychiatric effects—depression, suicidality and homicidal ideation. Also exercise caution in those with diabetes and operating heavy machinery.

Note: Recently, combination patch and gum has been approved for over-the counter use in Canada. Details can be found on the label of the product.

*(Cahill et al., 2010; Hughes et al., 2007; Stead et al., 2008; Fiore et al., 2008)

Pharmacotherapy has evidence in those who smoke 10 or more cigarettes per day and in those interested in stopping smoking. Note that treatment is for eight to 12 weeks and success is defined as not smoking at the six-month or more follow-up time point from the quit attempt or at least three months after the medication is stopped. The actual duration of treatment needs to be individualized.

Psychoeducation

Patients and their families or caregivers should be counselled about the nature of addiction. Specifically they should be helped to understand that:
· Addiction is a disease process that is amenable to treatment.
· Addiction is a chronic, relapsing, remitting condition and single episodes of treatment rarely lead to a permanent remission.
· Patients must be ready for change to accept advice.
· Exploration of the factors contributing to substance use rather than lecturing is more effective.
· If the person is not ready to change, the role of families/caregivers is to support the person and not enable continued use.

What is reasonable to expect of a primary care clinician?

The five As

The World Health Organization describes the five As as:

> … a sequential series of steps to use during health care interactions, which facilitate patient-centred care and patient self-management. They represent an approach that emphasizes collaborative goal setting, patient skill-building to overcome barriers, self-monitoring, personalized feedback, and systematic links to community resources.

> They are *not* psychological counselling but a set of "how-to guidelines" for the entire health care team to use. (WHO, 2010)

The five As, adapted specifically for smoking cessation (Fiore et al., 2009), but with broad applicability to other substance use disorders, are the following:

Ask   Screen for substance use disorders.

Advise   Provide brief advice for patients presenting with an addiction-related complaint and offer harm reduction for those not ready to quit.

Assess   Re-evaluate the patient's stage of change at every appointment.

Assist   When they are ready to address their addiction, provide patients with support and intervention strategies.

Arrange   Be aware of community resources and refer to a specialist when necessary.

When to refer to a specialist

· For diagnostic clarification
· If the severity or complexity of the presentation is beyond the expertise of the family physician
· If the patient requires support and services provided by a specialized centre (e.g., pregnant women, trauma victims, youth)
· If there are multiple problems that could benefit from multidisciplinary case management
· If there is only a partial response or no response to treatment

Community and online resources

Resources for physicians

· U.S. Department of Health and Human Services and SAMHSA National Clearing House for Alcohol and Drug Information: www.ncadi.samhsa.gov
· U.S. Department of Health and Human Services, *Treating Tobacco Use and Dependence: 2008 Update. Quick Reference Guide for Clinicians*: www.ahrq.gov/clinic/tobacco/tobaqrg.pdf
· Motivational Interviewing: www.motivationalinterview.org
· Rethinking Stop-Smoking Medications: Myths and Facts (Ontario Medical

Association, 2008): www.oma.org/Health/tobacco/stopsmoke.asp
· Canadian Society of Addiction Medicine (CSAM): www.csam.org
· National Institute on Drug Abuse: www.nida.nih.gov

Resources for patients

MUTUAL AID GROUPS
· Alcoholics Anonymous: www.alcoholics-anonymous.org and
  www.aacanada.com
· Al-Anon Information Services/Alateen, 1-888-4AL-ANON
  (1-888-425-2666): www.al-anon.alateen.org
· Cocaine Anonymous: www.ca.org

HOTLINES
· Motherisk Alcohol and Substance Abuse Helpline: 1-877-FAS-INFO
  (327-4636)

RESOURCES FOR BOTH PATIENTS AND PHYSICIANS
· Centre for Addiction and Mental Health: www.camh.net

References

Butt, P., Beirness, D., Cesa, F., Gliksman, L., Paradis, C. & Stockwell. T.
(2010). *Alcohol and Health in Canada: A Summary of Evidence and Guidelines
for Low-Risk Drinking*. Prepared for the National Alcohol Strategy Advisory
Committee. Ottawa: Canadian Centre on Substance Abuse (CCSA).

Cahill, K., Stead, L.F. & Lancaster, T. (2010). Nicotine receptor partial
agonists for smoking cessation. *Cochrane Database of Systematic Reviews, 12*,
CD006103.

Fiore, M.C., Jaén, C.R., Baker, T.B., Bailey, W.C., Benowitz, N., Curry, S.J.
et al. (2008). *Treating Tobacco Use and Dependence: 2008 Update. Clinical
Practice Guideline*. Rockville, MD: U.S. Department of Health and Human
Services, Public Health Service. Retrieved from www.surgeongeneral.gov/
tobacco/treating_tobacco_use08.pdf

Fiore, M.C., Jaén, C.R., Baker, T.B., Bailey, W.C., Benowitz, N., Curry, S.J. et al. (2009). *Treating Tobacco Use and Dependence: 2008 Update. Quick Reference Guide for Clinicians*. Rockville, MD: U.S. Department of Health and Human Services. Public Health Service.

Hughes, J.R., Stead, L.F. & Lancaster, T. (2007). Antidepressants for smoking cessation. *Cochrane Database of Systematic Reviews, 1*, CD000031.

Selby, P. & Handford, C. (2010). Assessment of patients with substance-related disorders. In D.S. Goldbloom (Ed.), *Psychiatric Clinical Skills* (Rev. 1st ed.; pp. 147–165). Toronto: Centre for Addiction and Mental Health, pp. 147–165.

Stead, L.F., Perera, R., Bullen, C., Mant, D. & Lancaster, T. (2008). Nicotine replacement therapy for smoking cessation. *Cochrane Database of Systematic Reviews, 1*, CD000146.

Sullivan, J.T., Sykora, K., Schneiderman, J., Naranjo, C.A. & Sellers, E.M. (1989). Assessment of alcohol withdrawal: The revised Clinical Institute Withdrawal Assessment for Alcohol scale (CIWA-Ar). *British Journal of Addiction, 84*, 1353-1357. Available from http://knowledgex.camh.net/primary_care/toolkits/addiction_toolkit/alcohol/Documents/Toolkit-Tool_CIWA.pdf

World Health Organization. (2010). *The 5 As*. Retrieved from http://www.who.int/diabetesactiononline/about/fiveAs/en/index.html

7

The patient who is psychotic

GEORGE FOUSSIAS AND Z. JEFF DASKALAKIS

Schizophrenia and related psychotic disorders are chronic illnesses characterized by significant morbidity and mortality. This results as a consequence of the constellation of their psychiatric symptoms, as well as associated comorbid somatic illnesses including diabetes mellitus, obesity, metabolic syndrome, hypertension and cardiovascular and pulmonary disease. These arise as a result of disease-related factors (e.g., the impact of symptoms on help-seeking behaviour), lifestyle factors (e.g., increased rates of cigarette smoking, poor diet and inactivity), effects of antipsychotic treatment, and reduced access to primary medical care. This complex interplay between psychiatric symptoms and somatic illness highlights the importance of ongoing collaborative multidisciplinary care in the treatment of individuals with schizophrenia and related disorders.

Differential diagnosis

- Organic conditions (see page 117)
- Delirium or dementia (see also chapter 10)
- Substance intoxication or withdrawal (see also chapter 6)
- Mood disorder with psychotic features (depression or mania)

Mood disorder with psychotic features can be differentiated from schizophrenia by the exclusive appearance of psychotic symptoms during periods of mood disturbance.

Brief psychotic disorder

Brief psychotic disorder is characterized by psychotic symptoms lasting at least one day but less than one month.

Schizophreniform disorder

Schizophreniform disorder is characterized by symptoms of schizophrenia that last at least one month but less than six months.

Delusional disorder

Delusional disorder is characterized by non-bizarre delusions and the absence of other characteristic symptoms of schizophrenia (e.g., hallucinations, negative symptoms, disorganized speech or behaviour).

Schizoaffective disorder

Schizoaffective disorder is characterized by a mood episode that is concurrent with psychotic symptoms of schizophrenia, where the mood symptoms are present for a substantial portion of the total duration of the disturbance, and psychotic symptoms must also be present for at least two weeks in the absence of prominent mood symptoms (see page 116 for DSM diagnostic criteria).

Schizophrenia

Schizophrenia is characterized by the presence of symptoms (e.g., hallucinations, delusions, negative symptoms, disorganized speech or behaviour) for at least six months (see page 115 for DSM diagnostic criteria).

How to make the diagnosis in less than five minutes (rapid assessment)

Quick screening questions for psychotic symptoms include:
- Have you had any strange or odd experiences lately that you can't explain?
- Do you ever hear things that other people can't hear, such as noises, or the voices of other people whispering or talking?

- Do you ever have visions or see things that other people can't see?
- Do you ever feel that people are bothering you or trying to harm you?
- Has it ever seemed like people were talking about you or taking special notice of you?
- Are you afraid of anything or anyone?

An answer of "yes" to any of these questions indicates the need for a more detailed assessment. In addition, it is always important to obtain corroborating information from caregivers or others close to the patient.

DSM-IV-TR Criteria for Schizophrenia

A. *Characteristic symptoms*: Two (or more) of the following, each present for a significant portion of time during a 1-month period (or less if successfully treated):

   (1) delusions

   (2) hallucinations

   (3) disorganized speech (e.g., frequent derailment or incoherence)

   (4) grossly disorganized or catatonic behaviour

   (5) negative symptoms, i.e., affective flattening, alogia, or avolition

   Note: Only one Criterion A symptom is required if delusions are bizarre or hallucinations consist of a voice keeping up a running commentary on the person's behaviour or thoughts, or two or more voices conversing with each other.

B. *Social/occupational dysfunction*: For a significant portion of the time since the onset of the disturbance, one or more major areas of functioning such as work, interpersonal relations, or self-care are markedly below the level achieved prior to the onset (or when the onset is in childhood or adolescence, failure to achieve expected level of interpersonal, academic, or occupational achievement).

C. *Duration*: Continuous signs of the disturbance persist for at least 6 months. This 6-month period must include at least 1 month of symptoms (or less if successfully treated) that meet Criterion A (i.e., active-phase symptoms) and may include periods of prodromal or residual symptoms. During these prodromal or residual periods, the signs of the disturbance may be manifested by only negative symptoms or two or more symptoms listed in Criterion A present in an attenuated form (e.g., odd beliefs, unusual perceptual experiences).

D. *Schizoaffective and Mood Disorder exclusion*: Schizoaffective Disorder and Mood Disorder With Psychotic Features have been ruled out because either (1) no Major Depressive, Manic, or Mixed Episodes have occurred concurrently with the active-phase symptoms; or (2) if mood episodes have occurred during active-phase symptoms, their total duration has been brief relative to the duration of the active and residual periods.

E. *Substance/general medical condition exclusion*: The disturbance is not due to the direct physiological effects of a substance (e.g., a drug of abuse, a medication) or a general medical condition.

F. *Relationship to a Pervasive Developmental Disorder*: If there is a history of Autistic Disorder or another Pervasive Developmental Disorder, the additional diagnosis of Schizophrenia is made only if prominent delusions or hallucinations are also present for at least a month (or less if successfully treated).

Reprinted with permission from the *Diagnostic and Statistical Manual of Mental Disorders*, Fourth Edition, Text Revision (Copyright 2000). American Psychiatric Association.

DSM-IV-TR Criteria for Schizoaffective Disorder

A. An uninterrupted period of illness during which, at some time, there is either a Major Depressive Episode, a Manic Episode, or a Mixed Episode concurrent with symptoms that meet Criterion A for Schizophrenia.

Note: The Major Depressive Episode must include Criterion A1: depressed mood.

B. During the same period of illness, there have been delusions or hallucinations for at least 2 weeks in the absence of prominent mood symptoms.

C. Symptoms that meet criteria for a mood episode are present for a substantial portion of the total duration of the active and residual periods of the illness.

D. The disturbance is not due to the direct physiological effects of a substance (e.g., a drug of abuse, a medication) or a general medical condition.

Specify type:

Bipolar Type: if the disturbance includes a Manic or a Mixed Episode
(or a Manic or a Mixed Episode and Major Depressive Episodes)

Depressive Type: if the disturbance only includes Major Depressive Episodes

Reprinted with permission from the *Diagnostic and Statistical Manual of Mental Disorders*,
Fourth Edition, Text Revision (Copyright 2000). American Psychiatric Association.

How to reasonably rule out underlying organic pathology

Many medical illnesses can cause psychotic symptoms, but they generally
have other symptoms and signs associated with the primary disease.

For first presentations of psychosis, a physical examination including
a neurological examination, a general medical history and review of symptoms should be conducted. Unless otherwise indicated by the history and/
or physical examination, screening blood tests should include complete
blood count, blood chemistry including electrolytes, liver function tests,
and thyroid stimulating hormone test.

A toxicology screen is also recommended as substance intoxication and
withdrawal can also present with psychotic symptoms.

In addition, for individuals presenting for the first time with psychotic symptoms a CT or MRI is recommended to rule out structural brain abnormalities.

Treatment options

The following section will focus on the treatment of psychotic symptoms
in the context of schizophrenia or schizoaffective disorder. The same general
principles apply for the treatment of psychosis in the context of other illnesses; however the underlying illness must be addressed (e.g., psychosis
in the context of delirium, major depressive episode with psychotic features).

Psychopharmacology

ACUTE TREATMENT

The goals for acute treatment of a patient presenting with psychosis include:
· diagnostic assessment
· assessment of the potential for danger to self or others
· engagement of the patient and caregivers in the treatment process, including a discussion around risks and benefits of treatment
· initiation of pharmacologic treatment as soon as possible.

The goal of treatment is full remission of symptoms and return to baseline function. Second-generation antipsychotic medications (SGAs) are the first-choice treatments, particularly for previously unmedicated patients who are particularly sensitive to acute extrapyramidal and sedative side-effects caused by antipsychotics.

The SGAs—including olanzapine, risperidone, quetiapine, ziprasidone and aripiprazole—are all first-line medications and offer improved tolerability, particularly with regard to extrapyramidal symptoms, compared with first-generation antipsychotics (FGAs) (see Table 7.1 on page 120).

Usually there is not one definite choice of medication for any given patient, since there is much individual variability in efficacy and side-effects. The choice of antipsychotic is based primarily on individual profiles of efficacy and tolerability:
· All SGAs (except clozapine) appear to be equally effective in treatment of psychosis in schizophrenia, with some recent evidence suggesting the possibility of a slight advantage in effectiveness for olanzapine.
· There is also some emerging evidence that SGAs and FGAs may be equally effective in the treatment of schizophrenia or schizoaffective disorder.
· Clozapine appears to be a unique SGA that exhibits superiority in the treatment of treatment-resistant patients with schizophrenia or schizoaffective disorder (i.e., patients who have not benefited from previous trials of two antipsychotics).
· All antipsychotics carry a risk of extrapyramidal symptoms and tardive

dyskinesia, although the risk appears to be higher with FGAs compared to SGAs. Of the SGAs, the risk of extrapyramidal symptoms appears to be highest with risperidone.
- All antipsychotics carry a risk of weight gain and metabolic abnormalities, although the risk appears to be higher with SGAs, and in particular with olanzapine, quetiapine and clozapine.
- Risperidone is the SGA most commonly associated with elevated prolactin levels and subsequent amenorrhea and sexual dysfunction.
- Ziprasidone carries a potential risk of QTc prolongation, and as such is contraindicated in patients with a prolonged QTc interval.
- Clozapine treatment carries a risk of agranulocytosis, which requires regular monitoring of white blood cell and neutrophil counts (weekly for the first six months, biweekly for the next six months, and monthly thereafter). The risk is approximately 0.5 to two per cent, and appears to be greatest in the early stages of treatment initiation.
- In the case of schizoaffective disorder, treatment typically consists of a combination of an antipsychotic and medication aimed at treatment of the mood disturbance (see "The patient who is depressed" on page 13 and "The patient who is manic" on page 27).

MAINTENANCE TREATMENT
The goals for maintenance treatment of schizophrenia or schizoaffective disorder are:
- improvement in functional recovery
- prevention of relapse and recurrence
- maintenance of treatment adherence.

Discontinuing medications
Following treatment of a first episode of psychosis, with symptom remission and functional recovery while on medications for approximately two years, consideration may be given for a trial of no medications. There are, however, no predictive factors indicating which patients can safely and permanently discontinue antipsychotic medications. Withdrawal of antipsychotic medications should be done gradually over six to 12 months, with symptoms and functioning monitored closely during this time.

Table 7.1 First- and second-generation antipsychotic medications[1]

MEDICATION	STARTING DOSE (MG/DAY)	USUAL TARGET DOSE (MG/DAY)	MAXIMAL DOSAGE (MG/DAY)[2]	FREQUENCY
Second-generation antipsychotics — oral — generic name (brand name)				
Risperidone (Risperdal)	0.5–2	2–6	8	od or bid
Olanzapine (Zyprexa)	5–10	10–20	20	od
Quetiapine (Seroquel)	50–100	300–800	800	od or bid
Quetiapine XR (Seroquel XR)	300	400–800	800	od
Ziprasidone (Zeldox)[3]	80	120–160	200	bid with meals
Aripiprazole (Abilify)	10–15	10–30	30	od
Clozapine (Clozaril)	12.5–25	300–600	900	od to tid
Second-generation antipsychotics — depot — generic name (brand name)				
Risperidone long-acting injectable (Risperdal Consta)	12.5–25 (oral supple-mentation required for the first 3 weeks)	25–37.5	50	q2weeks

First-generation antipsychotics — oral — generic name (brand name)

Haloperidol (Haldol)	1–3	4–12	20	bid or tid
Fluphenazine (Moditen)	2.5–10	1–5	20	od to tid
Flupenthixol (Fluanxol)	1–3	3–6	12	tid
Perphenazine (Trilafon)	8–16	16–64	64	bid to qid
Loxapine (Loxapac)	10–50	60–100	250	bid to qid
Zuclopenthixol (Clopixol)	10–50	20–60	100	bid or tid

First-generation antipsychotics — depot — generic name (brand name)

Haloperidol decanoate (Haldol LA)	25	50–200	300	q4 weeks
Fluphenazine decanoate (Modecate)	2.5–12.5	12.5–50	100	q2–4 weeks
Flupenthixol decanoate (Fluanxol Depot)	5–20	20–80	80	q2–3 weeks
Zuclopenthixol acetate (Clopixol Acuphase)	25–50	50–150	400 (cumulative dose)	q2–3 days
Zuclopenthixol decanoate (Clopixol Depot)	100–200	150–300	400 q2weeks	q2–4 weeks

[1] Not an exhaustive list of all FGA or FGA-depot antipsychotics available. Dosages are for adult patients. In the elderly, appropriate dosage adjustments may be necessary.

[2] Based on *Compendium of Pharmaceuticals and Specialties* (Canadian Pharmacists Association, 2009) values, or when not available, *Clinical Handbook of Psychotropic Drugs*, 18th edition (Virani, et al., 2009).

[3] Ziprasidone must be taken with meals to ensure adequate medication absorption.

Relapse rates for patients off antipsychotic medications are estimated at 60 per cent or higher over two years. Of patients with a first episode of psychosis, 80 per cent are at risk of a second episode within the first three to five years, with recovery from subsequent episodes being slower and often less complete. Following a second psychotic episode, it becomes highly unlikely that patients will remain relapse-free in the future while off antipsychotic medication.

Inadequate response to pharmacotherapy

If response is inadequate, re-evaluate the following:
· the diagnosis
· treatment non-adherence (often due to poor insight into illness)
· substance use or abuse.

Pharmacological strategies for initial non-responders include:
· optimization of antipsychotic dose
· substitution with another antipsychotic medication
· substitution with a long-acting intramuscular depot antipsychotic medication (if treatment adherence is a factor).

After referral, a specialist may:
· prescribe clozapine for treatment-resistant patients who have shown partial or total non-response to previous trials of at least two other antipsychotic medications
· augment clozapine (e.g., lamotrigine, valproic acid)
· offer adjunctive electroconvulsive therapy (ECT).

Managing persistent negative symptons

Persistent negative symptoms are a frequent feature of schizophrenia or schizoaffective disorder, characterized by enduring affective flattening, poverty of speech, social withdrawal and amotivation. For these patients, it is important to evaluate whether these negative symptoms are a consequence of the underlying illness (i.e., primary) or, alternatively, are secondary to other causes including:

- residual paranoid delusions
- anxiety
- depression
- over-sedation
- antipsychotic-induced extrapyramidal symptoms
- antipsychotic-induced dysphoria.

There is limited evidence to support a benefit of SGAs over FGAs in the treatment of primary negative symptoms, although they may be somewhat better with respect to secondary negative symptoms attributable to extrapyramidal symptoms. Treatments of secondary negative symptoms through adjunctive medications or optimization of antipsychotic medication is important.

There are limited options for the treatment of primary negative symptoms at present. There is some evidence to suggest adjunctive antidepressant treatment with SSRIs may be of some benefit.

Avoiding drug–drug interactions

Numerous medications (e.g., psychotropic medications, antibiotics, antifungal agents) and natural products may impact hepatic metabolism through the cytochrome P450 (CYP 450) system, and thus interfere with antipsychotic medication metabolism.

- In a patient population characterized by a high rate of co-occurring cigarette smoking, the induction of the CYP 450 system, and in particular isoenzyme 1A2, can cause increased metabolism of some antipsychotic medications, including clozapine and olanzapine, thus requiring somewhat higher doses in these patients.
- Abrupt smoking cessation can cause a gradual reduction in metabolism of antipsychotic medications through CYP 1A2, with the gradual emergence of signs and symptoms of antipsychotic toxicity if antipsychotic dosages are not monitored and adjusted accordingly (especially with clozapine).
- Fluvoxamine can markedly inhibit CYP 1A2 and can increase blood levels of drugs that are metabolized primarily by this isoenzyme (caution is recommended in those patients treated with clozapine).

· Fluoxetine and paroxetine can inhibit CYP 2D6 and thus cause increased plasma levels for many antipsychotics that are metabolized through this isoenzyme (e.g., risperidone, aripiprazole, haloperidol, fluphenazine).
· Carbamazepine is a potent inducer of CYP 3A4 and thus can cause reduced plasma concentrations of several antipsychotics that are metabolized through this isoenzyme (e.g., quetiapine, ziprasidone).
· Ziprasidone is contraindicated in patients who are concurrently being treated with medications that can prolong the QT interval (e.g., quinidine, type Ia and II antiarrhythmics, certain antibiotics).

Psychotherapy and psychosocial interventions

Psychotherapy and psychosocial interventions are an important component of treatment for patients with schizophrenia or schizoaffective disorder, and are typically administered through local specialty psychiatric services and community treatment teams. These approaches include:
· cognitive-behavioural therapy (CBT), particularly for treatment-resistant patients with persistent positive and/or negative symptoms
· psychoeducation (see below)
· family interventions including family psychoeducation, multiple-family groups (particularly early in the course of the illness), and evaluating and addressing caregiver burden
· employment and academic interventions including supported employment and academic accommodations through student services at secondary and post-secondary institutions
· social skills and life skills training
· case management (e.g., community case worker/community treatment team for housing and employment assistance, Ontario Disability Support Program assistance).

PSYCHOEDUCATION
Psychoeducation aimed at increasing knowledge about a patient's illness should be an ongoing process with patients and their families.

Often the focus revolves around treatment non-adherence that can result from:
· lack of insight into their illness
· concurrent alcohol or other drug abuse
· problems with therapeutic alliance
· medication side-effects
· complicated dosage schedules
· problems accessing treatment
· financial obstacles to obtaining medication.

Use simple messages to improve adherence to medications:
· "Antipsychotics can take a couple of weeks to start working."
· "Take the medications every day."
· "Side-effects are usually mild and improve over time."
· "Continue on medications, even after feeling better, or symptoms may return."
· "Do not stop antipsychotic medication before checking with your doctor."
· "Alcohol and recreational drugs can affect how well the medication works."

Take a self-management approach:
· Always include patient education (e.g., patient information handouts).
· Involve patients, and their families when appropriate, in the management of their own illness by actively collaborating with them in the diagnosis and treatment planning.

Other treatments
Electroconvulsive therapy (ECT) may offer some benefit for treatment-resistant psychotic symptoms, in combination with antipsychotic medication. There is also some emerging evidence to suggest repetitive transcranial magnetic stimulation (rTMS) may benefit some patients with treatment-resistant psychotic symptoms.

What is reasonable to expect of a primary care clinician?

· Diagnosing and carrying out initial screening for underlying medical illnesses
· Assessing suicide risk (see "Assessment and management of suicide risk," page 237)
· Initiating treatment and monitoring treatment response and symptom severity
· Monitoring extrapyramidal symptoms
· Monitoring metabolic and cardiovascular risk factors for all patients prescribed antipsychotic medication, and in particular SGAs, regardless of which physician is prescribing antipsychotic medications (see Table 7.2 for recommended monitoring guidelines)
· Managing comorbid somatic illnesses
· Referring when necessary (see next section)

When to refer to a specialist

· First presentation of psychotic symptoms
· Diagnostic clarification and treatment
· Severe presentation (safety risks to self or others, serious functional impairment, comorbid medical or substance use issues)
· Refractory to standard treatment (two or more medication trials)
· Acute decompensation
· When considering the use of clozapine or ECT

Community resources

Medical supports:

· community mental health clinics or hospital-based psychiatry outpatient clinics
· university- or hospital-affiliated schizophrenia programs
Self-help or support groups:
· Canadian Mental Health Association: www.cmha.ca
· local support groups, see Schizophrenia Society of Canada: www.schizophrenia.ca

Table 7.2 Recommended monitoring guidelines[1]

CLINICAL AND LABORATORY MONITORING	MONITORING FREQUENCY	
	ACUTE PHASE	STABLE PHASE
Hematology: CBC	baseline	yearly
Blood chemistry: electrolytes, renal function, liver function, thyroid function	baseline	yearly
Cataracts: functional inquiry and ocular exam	baseline	q2 years to age 40, then yearly
Vital signs	baseline	as indicated clinically
ECG	as indicated clinically, and before starting antipsychotics with QTc effects	as indicated clinically
Extrapyramidal signs and symptoms: Parkinsonism, dystonia, dyskinesia, akathisia	baseline, when changing antipsychotic dose, then weekly for 2–4 weeks	q6 months and as needed
Body mass: BMI, waist circumference	baseline, then monthly for 6 months when starting antipsychotic	q3 months
Fasting blood sugar	baseline, and 4 months after starting a new antipsychotic	yearly, or more frequently if symptomatic or gaining weight
Fasting lipid panel	baseline	at least q2 years, q6 months if LDL elevated

Table 7.2 Recommended monitoring guidelines, continued

CLINICAL AND LABORATORY MONITORING	MONITORING FREQUENCY	
	ACUTE PHASE	STABLE PHASE
Endocrine and sexual function: functional inquiry and prolactin level where indicated	baseline, monthly for 3 months after starting new antipsychotic	yearly

[1] Based on Canadian Psychiatric Association Working Group (2005) and American Psychiatric Association (2000).

Community and online resources

Resources for primary care providers
· Canadian Psychiatric Association treatment guidelines: http://publications. cpa-apc.org/browse/documents/67
· National Institute for Health and Clinical Excellence treatment guidelines: http://guidance.nice.org.uk/CG82

Resources for patients and their families
· Canadian Mental Health Association: www.cmha.ca
· Schizophrenia Society of Canada: www.schizophrenia.ca

References
Butt, P., Beirness, D., Cesa, F., Gliksman, L., Paradis, C. & Stockwell. T. (2010). *Alcohol and Health in Canada: A Summary of Evidence and Guidelines for Low-Risk Drinking.* Prepared for the National Alcohol Strategy Advisory Committee. Ottawa: Canadian Centre on Substance Abuse (CCSA).

8

The patient with an eating disorder

DAVID S. GOLDBLOOM

Introduction

In a Canadian context of both increasing obesity and continuing cultural pressure to be thin—which affects predominantly women but increasingly men as well—dieting and disordered eating (unstructured meals, grazing, food fads, etc.) are common. Up to 80 per cent of adult women have dieted or are currently dieting. But while disordered eating is common, the formal eating disorders—anorexia nervosa, bulimia nervosa and binge eating disorder—are relatively rare, affecting one to three per cent of the female population.

However, the distress, physical complications and even mortality risks of these eating disorders require primary care providers to be vigilant in their diagnosis of people at risk. The scarcity of specialized treatment resources for people with eating disorders means primary care providers will inevitably be involved in the patient's care.

The secrecy and shame associated with having an eating disorder may conceal detection, and the negative attitudes some health professionals have toward people with eating disorders may compromise treatment. For all these reasons, the diagnosis and treatment of eating disorders in primary care remains an important responsibility, and at times a difficult challenge.

Clinical presentation

There are no other psychiatric disorders with as many physical signs and laboratory findings as the eating disorders. However, obesity is not one of those signs as most people who are overweight do not have a formal eating disorder. Rather, it is more likely the normal-weight or underweight woman who may present to you for help with an undiagnosed eating disorder. The chief complaint is rarely, "I think I have an eating disorder." Rather, she or he (up to 90 per cent of eating disorders occur in women) may ask for help with:

· constipation, bloating or fluid retention
· weight-loss advice despite being at normal weight
· problems with mood instability, anxiety, sleep or concentration difficulties.

Additionally, the patient may show some of these physical and laboratory findings:

· marked weight loss
· bradycardia and hypotension
· amenorrhea
· impaired temperature regulation
· acrocyanosis
· delayed gastric emptying
· hair loss, dry skin and growth of lanugo hair
· hypokalemic, hypochloremic metabolic alkalosis
· elevated salivary amylase
· parotid hypertrophy
· anemia
· EKG findings including low voltage, T wave inversion, prolonged QTc interval
· osteoporosis at a young age.

Screening for eating disorders in less than five minutes

A five-question screening test, similar to the CAGE screen for alcohol dependence, called the SCOFF questionnaire has been developed for eating disorders. The name is somewhat controversial because the acronym is defined as "greedy eating." The questionnaire has been evaluated and compared with other measures in specialty clinics and in primary care in both England and the United States. It has been adopted by most Primary Care Trusts in the United Kingdom. Because in the British version the "O" represents "one stone" of weight and "sick" is understood to be "vomit," the American version is provided below in more familiar language to Canadians.

The SCOFF questionnaire

1. Do you make yourself vomit (**S**ick) because you feel uncomfortably full?

2. Do you worry that you have lost **C**ontrol over how much you eat?

3. Have you recently lost more than 15 pounds (**O**ne stone) in a 3-month period?

4. Do you believe you are **F**at when others say you are too thin?

5. Would you say that **F**ood dominates your life?

Two or more positive answers to these questions constitute a positive SCOFF screen, with good sensitivity and specificity and minimal time or skill requirement for the physician or the patient.

Reproduced with permission from Morgan et al., 1999. Copyright 2010 BMJ Publishing Group Ltd.

Diagnosing eating disorders in primary care
See pages 133–135 for DSM criteria for eating disorders.

If a patient screens positive or you are simply clinically concerned, then you need to take time to explore, in a non-critical way, whether a formal eating disorder exists. This includes taking a comprehensive weight history and inquiring about body image, eating behaviours, purging behaviours, medical complications and psychiatric complications.

Weight history
Take a comprehensive lifetime weight history, including the following:
· current weight and height

Ask:

"How do you feel about this weight? At what weight do you feel fat?"

· highest and lowest adult weights.

QUESTIONS THAT WILL HELP CLARIFY TREATMENT GOALS AND
OBSTACLES

· Ideal weight — Ask: "How would your life be different at that weight?"
· Menstrual threshold weight — Target weight for treatment must be above
  this weight.
· Frequency and routine of weighing self — This part of the history will help
  the clinician to better understand how the eating disorder governs the life
  of the patient.

Body image
Ask the patient:
· "How do you see yourself currently?"
· "How much does your weight and shape determine how you feel about
  yourself as a person?"
· "Do you fear gaining even small amounts of weight?"

Eating behaviours
Ask the patient about:
· dieting history
· caloric and food group restrictions
· episodes of binge eating with a sense of loss of control and consumption
  of foods that are typically avoided.

Purging behaviours
Ask the patient about:
· self-induced vomiting
· use of laxatives, diuretics, diet pills
· intensive exercise for purposes of weight loss
· cigarette smoking to suppress appetite.

Medical complications
As listed previously (see "Clinical presentation," page 132).

Psychiatric complications
Determine if there are any other psychiatric complications, including:
· depression
· anxiety
· obsessionality
· impulsivity
· substance abuse.

DSM-IV-TR Criteria for Anorexia Nervosa

A. Refusal to maintain body weight at or above a minimally normal weight for age and height (e.g., weight loss leading to maintenance of body weight less than 85% of that expected; or failure to make expected weight gain during period of growth, leading to body weight less than 85% of expected).

B. Intense fear of gaining weight or becoming fat, even though underweight.

C. Disturbance in the way in which one's body weight or shape is experienced, undue influence of body weight or shape on self-evaluation, or denial of the seriousness of the current low body weight.

D. In postmenarcheal females, amenorrhea, i.e., the absence of at least three consecutive menstrual cycles. (A woman is considered to have amenorrhea if her periods occur only following hormone, e.g., estrogen, administration).

Specify type:

Restricting Type: during the current episode of Anorexia Nervosa, the person has not regularly engaged in binge-eating or purging behaviour (i.e., self-induced vomiting or the misuse of laxatives, diuretics or enemas)

Binge-Eating/Purging Type: during the current episode of Anorexia Nervosa, the person has regularly engaged in binge-eating or purging behaviour (i.e., self-induced vomiting or the misuse of laxatives, diuretics or enemas)

Reprinted with permission from the *Diagnostic and Statistical Manual of Mental Disorders*, Fourth Edition, Text Revision (Copyright 2000). American Psychiatric Association.

DSM-IV-TR Criteria for Bulimia Nervosa

A. Recurrent episodes of binge eating. An episode of binge eating is characterized by both of the following:

   1. eating, in a discrete period of time (e.g., within any 2-hour period), an amount of food that is definitely larger than most people would eat during a similar period of time and under similar circumstances

   2. a sense of lack of control over eating during the episode (e.g., a feeling that one cannot stop eating or control what or how much one is eating)

B. Recurrent inappropriate compensatory behaviour in order to prevent weight gain, such as self-induced vomiting; misuse of laxatives, diuretics, enemas, or other medications; fasting; or excessive exercise.

C. The binge eating and inappropriate compensatory behaviours both occur, on average, at least twice a week for 3 months.

D. Self-evaluation is unduly influenced by body shape and weight.

E. The disturbance does not occur exclusively during episodes of anorexia nervosa.

Specify type:

Purging Type: during the current episode of Bulimia Nervosa, the person has regularly engaged in self-induced vomiting or the misuse of laxatives, diuretics, or enemas

Nonpurging Type: during the current episode of Bulimia Nervosa, the person has used other inappropriate compensatory behaviours, such as fasting or excessive exercise, but has not regularly engaged in self-induced vomiting or the misuse of laxatives, diuretics, or enemas

Reprinted with permission from the *Diagnostic and Statistical Manual of Mental Disorders*, Fourth Edition, Text Revision (Copyright 2000). American Psychiatric Association.

DSM-IV-TR Criteria for Eating Disorder Not Otherwise Specified

The Eating Disorder Not Otherwise Specified category is for disorders of eating that do not meet criteria for any specific Eating Disorder. Examples include:

1. For females, all the criteria for Anorexia Nervosa are met except that the individual has regular menses.

2. All of the criteria for Anorexia Nervosa are met except that, despite significant weight loss, the individual's current weight is in the normal range.

3. All of the criteria for Bulimia Nervosa are met except that the binge eating and inappropriate compensatory mechanisms occur at a frequency of less than twice a week or for a duration of less than 3 months.

4. The regular use of inappropriate compensatory behaviour by an individual of normal body weight after eating small amounts of food (e.g., self-induced vomiting after the consumption of two cookies).

5. Repeatedly chewing and spitting out, but not swallowing, large amounts of food.

6. Binge eating disorder: recurrent episodes of binge eating in the absence of the regular use of inappropriate compensatory behaviours characteristic of Bulimia Nervosa.

Reprinted with permission from the *Diagnostic and Statistical Manual of Mental Disorders*, Fourth Edition, Text Revision (Copyright 2000). American Psychiatric Association.

Differential diagnosis

Because you are a primary care provider and not an eating disorders specialist, you also have the responsibility to rule out other causes of the clinical presentation. While people can lose weight for many reasons, the diagnosis of eating disorders requires the "nervosa" component—the undue preoccupation with body weight and shape, its influence on self-perception, and the morbid fear of becoming fat. The medical differential diagnosis includes:

· hyperthyroidism
· malignancy
· malabsorption
· inflammation (e.g., Crohn's disease, ulcerative colitis).

A careful history will rule out most of these possibilities, but a physical examination and some laboratory investigation will also help in clarifying the diagnosis and demonstrate your concern for your patient.

Other psychiatric disorders can be superficially mistaken for an eating disorder. These include:

· depression (accompanied by a true anorexia and weight loss)
· conversion disorder (belief that something is stuck in the throat and food cannot pass)
· schizophrenia (food avoidance based on the delusion that it is poisoned)
· substance abuse (psychostimulants that induce weight loss).

Again, a careful and sympathetic history will usually clarify the diagnosis. Further, your willingness to accept that the patient has an eating disorder will have a permissive effect on disclosure, since the patient has likely already made a diagnosis via the Internet.

For many health care providers, the seemingly conscious element of control in people with eating disorders is frustrating and even infuriating. It is important to understand that:

· While issues around seeking control may catapult someone into an eating disorder, the problem ends up controlling and dominating the person.

· While eating disorders cause numerous medical and psychiatric complications, they may also serve some adaptive function for patients (e.g., helping them to feel more in control; being praised for weight loss). If you find out what that function is, patients are more likely to feel that you "get" them as a person beyond their weight and their symptoms.

It is also important to meet and talk with the patient's family. In addition to providing collateral history, they will likely feel overwhelmed and worried and will need your support.

Treatment principles

Establish your role

Establish your role and responsibility for physical health as well as your relationship to other providers who may be involved.

Cultivate trust

While this may seem obvious for all patients, cultivating trust is particularly relevant in the context of treating eating disorders. You are asking someone to relinquish behaviours which, despite being maladaptive overall, serve some useful purpose; you are asking patients who may feel that much of their life is out of control to relinquish control over their weight and their eating behaviour. You will need to earn their trust.

Collaborate

Even though formal eating disorders services are scarce and have long waiting lists, you may need to enlist the help of a nutritionist or dietician to assist with meal planning, a counsellor or therapist to provide support and psychotherapy, and a consulting psychiatrist. If the family is involved, they should also be seen as collaborators with tremendous expertise in the life journey of the patient.

Treatment options

Psychoeducation

Although people with eating disorders may seem at first to have an encyclopedic knowledge of nutrition, it is frequently infused with mythology and morality. And, despite an intellectual awareness of eating disorders, patients may feel terribly alone and unique in their problems. There are many accounts of eating disorders and strategies for coping with them that patients and families can access and identify with. It can help people see the connections between the symptoms that actually bother them (trouble sleeping or concentrating, mood instability) and their eating disorder, which may increase motivation to get better.

Beyond informing and motivating people, there is now evidence that patient self-help books and guided self-help (regular meetings with the primary care provider) can make a difference, primarily with regard to binge eating disorder and, to a lesser extent, bulimia nervosa. The best of these books are:

- McCabe. R.I., McFarlane, T.L. & Olmsted, M.P. (2004). *The Overcoming Bulimia Workbook*. Oakland, CA: New Harbinger. (All authors Canadian!)
- Cooper, P. (2009). *Overcoming Bulimia Nervosa and Binge Eating: A Self-Help Guide Using Cognitive-Behavioural Techniques* (2nd ed.). New York: Basic Books.
- Fairburn, C.G. (1995). *Overcoming Binge Eating*. New York: Guilford Press.

In addition, books exist for families of adolescents with eating disorders, such as:

- Katzman, D.K. & Pinhas, L. (2005). *Help for Eating Disorders: A Parent's Guide to Symptoms, Causes and Treatments*. Toronto: Robert Rose. (From the Hospital for Sick Children.)
- Lock, J. & Le Grange, D. (2005). *Help Your Teenager Beat an Eating Disorder*. New York: Guilford Press.

Monitoring and nutrition

You can play a key role not only in monitoring for progress and complications but also in liberating people from the tyranny of bathroom scales. You should assume responsibility for regular monitoring of weight and have the patient (and often reluctant family) throw out the home's scale. This makes weighing less frequent and patients less able to regulate their self-esteem and self-appraisal by minor fluctuations in weight. For the underweight patient, you need to establish a healthy weight range (not a single number because weight naturally fluctuates) that can be maintained without undue dieting and that will allow a return of regular menses.

Similarly, simply asking patients to keep a regular diary of their eating and associated behaviour can be both informative and transformative. It tells you what actually goes on, and the patients begin to see the connections between food, weight, emotions, thoughts and behaviours. Many of the self-help books provide templates for this kind of self-monitoring.

Restoring regular eating is an important therapeutic goal. Patients who feel a "good day" is one where they have not "given in" to hunger during the day are far more likely to binge eat at night, perpetuating the cycle of restriction and loss of control. Realizing that their fear of gaining significant weight from a single meal is not realistic will help reduce the anxiety about eating and the fear that it will become a runaway train.

A rate of weight gain of 0.5 – 1.0 kg per week is appropriate in anorexia nervosa when moving toward a target weight range.

Psychotherapy

Cognitive-behavioural therapy (CBT) and interpersonal therapy (IPT) are the most validated treatments for bulimia nervosa and binge eating disorder. However, many primary care providers — and some psychiatrists — may feel insufficiently skilled in these modalities. At the same time, training in these approaches is becoming more popular as continuing education. CBT is particularly appealing because it takes a common-sense, here-and-now approach, requires patients to do homework and challenge their own assumptions, and is explicitly focused on behavioural change. It is a skill set that can also be effective in the primary care management of depression, anxiety, irritable bowel syndrome and insomnia. Alternatively, community-based social workers, psychologists, occupational therapists and counsellors with this skill could be enlisted to the treatment team.

For anorexia nervosa, despite its recognition almost 150 years ago (the first reported case in Canada was in 1895) and its significant mortality, the evidence base for psychotherapy — or other treatments — is much weaker. There is a role for family therapy after weight restoration in adolescents.

Pharmacotherapy: Anorexia nervosa

For anorexia nervosa, the drug of choice is food. In sufficient quantities over enough time, it will reverse virtually all of the numerous laboratory and physical anomalies associated with the disorder. Equally important, it will reverse some of the psychiatric symptoms, such as mood instability, anxiety, impaired concentration and sleep disturbance.

You should resist the temptation to use antidepressants for the mood disturbance because there is no evidence for their effectiveness in the underweight state.

For some patients, the anticipatory anxiety before an appropriate meal can be so overwhelming that short-acting benzodiazepines are used (e.g., lorazepam), but there is no high-quality evidence beyond clinical experience to support the use of benzodiazepines.

The seemingly delusional body image distortion is not responsive to antipsychotic medication. Drugs that induce weight gain as a side-effect or drugs identified as appetite stimulants should not be used; available evidence shows they do not work. However, for weight-recovered people with anorexia nervosa, given their long-term vulnerability to mood and anxiety disorders, they may require subsequent pharmacotherapy.

Pharmacotherapy: Bulimia nervosa

There is a significant body of evidence regarding the efficacy of antidepressants in bulimia nervosa. In Canada, fluoxetine is the only such drug approved by Health Canada for the treatment of bulimia nervosa, and the dose at which people typically respond is 60 mg per day in a single dose (of note, 20 mg per day, often effective in depression, was no different than placebo in a major clinical trial in bulimia nervosa). In the published literature, there is no evidence of increased suicidality with fluoxetine for this disorder. Common side-effects include sleep disturbance and decreased sexual desire and function.

For binge eating disorder, there is evidence of moderate strength for the efficacy with a variety of SSRI antidepressants (fluoxetine, fluvoxamine, sertraline, citalopram), with greater reductions in binge eating and other psychiatric symptoms than placebo. However, dropout rates and placebo response rates were high.

When to refer to a specialist

There is limited availability of community and institutional resources for people with eating disorders — either individual clinicians or specialized programs. Nevertheless, you can look for such resources through the National Eating Disorder Information Centre (www.nedic.ca), a superb Canadian website with valuable information on supports and services both online and across the country, as well as articles and other information for health professionals, patients and families.

If there is diagnostic uncertainty, especially concerning possible comorbid psychiatric diagnoses, a psychiatric consultation should be obtained.

Note that:
· In anorexia nervosa, when weight loss becomes precipitous and out of control or reaches frank emaciation, hospitalization is usually required both to minimize the multiple physical complications and to provide intensive and supervised re-feeding.

· In bulimia nervosa, hospitalization is rarely required unless there is severe metabolic instability, electrolyte disturbance with cardiac risk from hypokalemia, or suicidality.
· In binge eating disorder, there is no current role for hospitalization.

It is important to think broadly about the term "specialist" when seeking treatment for this clinical population. People with specialized expertise may be found within primary care, pediatrics, internal medicine, women's health, nursing, psychology, nutrition, social work and occupational therapy. Additionally, community-based support groups for both patients and their families may provide specialized experiential expertise.

While caring for these patients can be challenging, the rewards of seeing their recovery are gratifying—and there is reason for optimism based on long-term outcome studies. A recent study of a primary-care-based cohort of patients with eating disorders showed that after four years of follow-up, 57 per cent of those initially diagnosed with anorexia nervosa and 61 per cent of those initially diagnosed with bulimia nervosa were recovered.

You are strongly encouraged to take a team-based approach using the available resources within your community. Such an approach helps your patient in meeting broad needs and helps you in shouldering the responsibility.

Community and online resources

· National Eating Disorder Information Centre (www.nedic.ca). This website provides extensive information about resources across Canada, highly relevant reading material, and access to the Cochrane library of systematic reviews of treatment interventions in eating disorders.
· Sheena's Place (www.sheenasplace.org). This community-based support centre for people with eating disorders and their families in Toronto provides extensive online resources.

References

Hill, L.S., Reid, F., Morgan, J.F. & Lacey, J.H. (2010). SCOFF, the development of an eating disorder screening questionnaire. *International Journal of Eating Disorders, 43* (4), 344–351. DOI:10.1002/eat.20679

Morgan, J.F., Reid, F. & Lacey, J.H. (1999). The SCOFF questionnaire: A new screening tool for eating disorders. *British Medical Journal, 319*, 1467–1468.

National Institute for Health and Clinical Excellence. (2004, January). *Core Interventions in the Treatment and Management of Anorexia Nervosa, Bulimia Nervosa and Related Eating Disorders* (Clinical Guideline 9). Retrieved from www.nice.org.uk/CG9

van Son, G.E., van Hoeken, D., van Furth, E.F., Donker, G.A. & Hoek HW. (2010). Course and outcome of eating disorders in a primary care-based cohort. *International Journal of Eating Disorders, 43* (2), 130–138. DOI: 10.1002/eat.20676

Williams, P.M., Goodie, J. & Motsinger, C.D. (2008). Treating eating disorders in primary care. *American Family Physician, 77* (2), 187–195.

9
The patient with
a personality disorder

MICHAEL ROSENBLUTH

Introduction

There are many kinds of difficult patients in primary care. These include those with complex medical diagnoses, refractory chronic conditions and personality problems that complicate treatment. This chapter will focus on the difficult patient with a personality disorder.

Patients with personality disorders are difficult to treat and frustrate their caregivers. Yet clinical experience, and recent signals from the literature, indicates that careful assessment and treatment can result in more positive outcomes than previously assumed (Zanarini et al., 2004).

This chapter will describe what a personality disorder is. The focus will be on borderline personality disorder because these patients are often seen in primary care settings and are often the most challenging to treat. The chapter will also provide an overview of diagnosis and treatment issues that are relevant in primary care. Lastly, the chapter will also review the role of co-ordinating the care of these patients to optimize outcomes and to avoid medico-legal issues.

Diagnostic issues

A person with a personality disorder is someone who has a deep-seated maladaptive style as part of his or her personality.

It is important that the maladaptive personality style be pervasive and long-standing from teenage years onward.

Axis I conditions

If, according to the history from patients or their families, the onset of the personality difficulties are recent, then the clinician must consider whether a DSM Axis I diagnosis may be the correct diagnosis.

It is important to distinguish between a personality disorder and an Axis I condition. Axis I conditions include:
· Major Depressive Disorder
· Generalized Anxiety Disorder
· Panic Disorder
· Posttraumatic Stress Disorder.

Sometimes, these conditions can cause patients to appear to have a personality disorder. When people are depressed, it can bring out the worst in their personality. They may appear to be someone with a personality disorder as they become more demanding, inappropriately persistent, emotionally reactive and irritable.

ONSET
Recent onset, rather than long-standing personality difficulties, suggest these characteristics are more reflective of an Axis I state than a personality disorder.

Thus, if it is not a chronic, long-standing issue from teenage years onward, but more circumscribed and following the development of an Axis I state, (e.g., Major Depressive Disorder or Generalized Anxiety Disorder), then diagnostically this is best considered as an Axis I condition and not a personality disorder. It is important to keep in mind that when patients have a remission from their Axis I condition or state, they no longer appear to be personality-disordered.

Some patients may look personality-disordered when they are dealing with characteristic stressors that are difficult for them. However, when the history taken from the patient or the people in his or her support system indicates that the maladaptive behaviours are limited to a response to the difficult stressors, then it is not a personality disorder.

Thus, it is important to have collateral history from family members or significant others regarding the chronicity of the behaviours. As well, patients can themselves describe what they were like before the Axis I condition (i.e., depression, hypomania or generalized anxiety state) set in. Lastly, when the state improves, you can see the change in the personality presentation.

Personality disorders

There are 10 personality disorders in the DSM-IV. They have a varying degree of research supporting their diagnosis. The most commonly diagnosed personality disorders are antisocial personality disorder and borderline personality disorder. Another personality disorder that primary care providers sometimes find difficult to diagnose and treat is narcissistic personality disorder.

Borderline personality disorder

When considering borderline personality disorder, the diagnosis must fulfil five out of nine criteria. These can best be recalled by the mnemonic

IMPULSIVE:
· **I**mpulsiveness in two potentially damaging areas (e.g., sex, substance use, shopping)
· **M**ood instability due to marked reactivity
· **P**aranoia or dissociation under stress
· **U**nstable self-image

· Labile intense relationships
· Suicidal gestures
· Inappropriate anger
· Vulnerability to abandonment, frantic efforts to avoid real or imagined abandonment
· Emptiness, chronic feelings of emptiness.

Narcissistic personality disorder

Patients with a narcissistic personality disorder are those who have chronic, maladaptive and persistent personality styles characterized by a pervasive pattern of grandiosity, a need for admiration and a lack of empathy beginning by early adulthood and presenting in a variety of contexts.

At least five of the following need to be present:
· grandiose sense of self-importance
· preoccupation with fantasies of unlimited success, power and brilliance, believing that he or she is special and unique and can only be understood by or associate with other special or high-status people
· need for excessive admiration and sense of entitlement
· interpersonally exploitive behaviour (i.e., takes advantage of others to achieve his or her ends)
· lack of empathy
· envy of others or belief that others are envious of him or her; arrogance
· exhibiting haughty behaviours or attitudes.

Frances (2005) has indicated that in supportive therapy it is important to "go with the flow." That is, it is important to admire the narcissistic patient, to provide information to the obsessive-compulsive patient, or to allow and maintain a distance from the schizoid patient.

Each of these strategies meets the patient's needs and supports necessary defences. Trying to change personality in individuals with long-standing character structure is a more challenging task that most primary care providers will be willing to defer.

Co-occuring Axis I disorders

Patients with personality disorders frequently have co-occurring Axis I diagnoses. In borderline personality disorder there is considerable research demonstrating that co-occurring Axis I disorders are extremely frequent. Zanarini et al. (1998) have indicated in a prospective, well-designed study that 96 per cent of patients with borderline personality disorder will have a lifetime Axis I comorbidity for mood disorders (including nine per cent comorbidity with bipolar disorder), 88 per cent with anxiety disorders and 55 per cent with posttraumatic stress disorders, 53 per cent with eating disorders and 64 per cent with substance abuse disorders.

Given this high comorbidity, the challenge in working with these patients is not only to identify and optimally manage their personality disorder but also to not overlook comorbid Axis I diagnoses. Primary care providers may find the Axis I diagnoses easier to deal with. Certainly patients with both Axis I and Axis II problems need treatment plans that address both the Axis I and the Axis II conditions.

Treatment prospects

Follow-up research has indicated that patients with borderline personality disorder can improve with treatment. Zanarini's group in 2004 indicated that on six-year follow-up over half the patients no longer met borderline personality disorder diagnostic criteria. Interestingly, they note that those patients who no longer met borderline personality disorder diagnostic criteria had a substantial decline in the comorbid Axis I traits described above. Those patients who met borderline personality disorder diagnostic criteria on six-year follow-up did not have a reduction of comorbid Axis I diagnoses (Zanarini et al., 2004).

There is controversy regarding whether this indicates that treating the personality disorder decreases the rates of co-occurring Axis I disorders or vice versa. The practical point for primary care providers is that all patients with personality disorder should be screened for comorbid Axis I diagnoses. These diagnoses should be treated robustly. This study and others with similar positive outcome findings are very encouraging. With proper diagnosis, treatment and time, a majority of these patients will "outgrow" their border-line personality disorder condition.

Making the Axis I diagnosis with co-occuring personality disorder

Clinicians often overlook the comorbid Axis I diagnoses. The typically chaotic presentation of patients with personality disorder — and clinicians' reactions to them — make the careful assessment of Axis I diagnoses difficult. Overlooking Axis I diagnoses diminishes the capacity to use the appropriate pharmacotherapy and psychotherapy to help alleviate the Axis I condition.

Sometimes these patients elicit a response of frustration in the clinician that contributes to overlooking a careful review of the longitudinal history and the clarification of the Axis I diagnosis. Again, this diminishes the treatment options available. Frustration may arise, for example, if a patient presents and is very difficult and disruptive in the waiting room, threatens self-harm and has a history of being emotionally reactive, responding to slights with self-harm and impulsive behaviours.

The clinician should clarify the presence of a personality disorder versus an Axis I diagnosis. One strategy for clarifying the presentation is by reviewing whether or not the patient has a long-standing history of negative maladaptive behaviours, or if these behaviours are restricted to when the Axis I diagnosis began.

It is important to clarify if those patients who appear personality disordered are really personality disordered or are individuals who have a refractory depression that is bringing out the worst in the patient's premorbid personality. It is important to remember that our clinical assessments tend to be cross-sectional whereas personality disorder requires a longitudinal review of functioning as indicated. A depressive state may colour patients' presentation making them look more personality-disordered than they are.

It is best to defer a personality assessment until the acute Axis I disorder has been successfully treated. Ask the patients to describe their personality prior to their depression. Get a collateral history from other members of the family or significant others who can confirm whether or not the maladaptive behaviours occur exclusively in the context of an Axis I diagnostic state, or are long-standing from childhood. Keep in mind that no matter how characterological the presentation, the diagnosis is unlikely to be a personality disorder if there is no supportive evidence from earlier in life.

Treatment issues

If the clinician confirms that there is long-standing personality pathology, it should not be a reason to avoid robust psychotherapy and/or pharmacotherapy. There have been several careful reviews of the literature that indicate that personality pathology, despite popular belief, does not worsen the outcome of the major depressive disorder (Mulder, 2002; Kool et al., 2005).

This is very important for primary care providers to keep in mind. The strongest support that personality pathology predicts poor outcome comes from the weakest studies, which did not carefully define personality, who was treated, how the treatment was conducted or how outcome was defined.

Treatment when there are co-occuring Axis I diagnoses

It is important to identify the comorbid Axis I diagnosis and treat robustly with the appropriate medication. If there is a comorbid personality disorder present, the main pharmacotherapy adjustment is to consider the toxicity of large amounts of medication, as patients with borderline personality disorder have a potential for overdose.

If there is comorbid bipolar disorder and borderline personality disorder, the use of lithium is somewhat controversial. There are several good studies that demonstrate that lithium for patients with bipolar disorder without comorbid personality disorder can reduce suicidal behaviours and completed suicides (Cipriani et al., 2005; Baldessarini et al., 2006). However, there is no research regarding suicide and the use of lithium in patients who have borderline personality disorder and comorbid bipolar disorder. This is important as lithium has a narrow therapeutic range regarding lethal overdose.

The comorbidity of bipolar disorder and borderline personality disorder has been suggested as anywhere from nine per cent (Zanarini et al., 2004) to 24 to 28 per cent (Gunderson et al., 2006). It is important to clarify this issue as modifications in pharmacotherapy (e.g., using atypical antipsychotics instead of lithium) will be required in those patients who have comorbid bipolar disorder with their borderline personality disorder.

When using medication, it is preferable to target identifiable comorbid Axis I diagnoses and use the appropriate medication indicated. However, when clear-cut comorbid Axis I diagnoses are not present, it is reasonable to consider medications for target symptoms (e.g., the tendency to have brief psychotic reactions or to be emotionally labile). There are signals from the literature that mood stabilizers (Cowdry, 1992) and atypical neuroleptics can help these target symptoms. Atypical neuroleptics have sometimes been seen as ego or brain "glue," making these patients less sensitive to the characteristic meltdowns that they are prone to.

Psychotherapies

There are many different kinds of psychotherapy that can be considered for this population. For primary care providers, the main issue is often whether or not the clinician has the time, interest or training to do psychotherapy, or can make a referral for these patients.

Dialectical behavioural therapy

Dialectical behavioural therapy (DBT) is the most researched psychotherapy for patients with borderline personality disorder. A form of cognitive-behavioural therapy, DBT emphasizes validation and acceptance of the patients, while focusing on change. DBT views these patients as having temperamental irregularities that in combination with an invalidating environment results in affective dysregulation (Linehan, 1992).

The goal of DBT is to learn functional strategies to modulate the reactivity, intensity and duration of patient reactions to stress. The focus is on validating the "kernel of truth." In reviewing when patients have their characteristic meltdowns, the clinician searches for what the trigger and motivation were for their response (i.e., the kernel of truth) which might be expressed as: "you wanted to escape the pain."

Busy primary care clinicians may not have the training or interest in using DBT or the other therapeutic modalities that psychotherapists may consider for working with these patients. However, primary care providers should be aware that they are uniquely situated to make a contribution to the care of these patients.

Primary care providers can help patients with personality disorders learn how to develop the "owner's manual" so they can better understand their personality. Patients need to look at how their core vulnerabilities can be managed. Primary care providers can make a difference by helping patients understand and manage their reactivity. They can help patients to understand the following points that make up the mnemonic TAACO:
· the **T**riggers that cause the emotional over-reactivity
· the **A**ntecedents that make those things the triggers (e.g., why did the boss's criticism trigger such a reaction and what might that reflect from earlier in life?)
· how the triggering situation could have been **A**nticipated so that it could have been better managed
· the **C**onsequences of the over-reaction
· the **O**ption that could have been used to avoid the reaction and the negative consequences.

Co-ordinating care

The APA guidelines on borderline personality disorder (APA, 2001) point out the importance of co-ordinating treatment provided by multiple clinicians. It is important to emphasize clear role definitions, what will occur when there is a crisis and that there should be some regular communication among clinicians and documentation thereof. It is important to determine which clinician is assuming primary or overall responsibility.

Often patients with personality disorders are attending other clinicians for therapy while attending the primary care physician for medication. It is important for primary care providers to be aware of any treatment the patient is receiving elsewhere, regardless of whether the patient was referred from primary care. This is because different therapies may inadvertently promote regression. Different therapies place greater value on uncovering early trauma and difficult emotional experiences. Sometimes this is necessary. Other times this occurs before the patient is ready to do that kind of therapeutic work.

The main point for primary care providers is that if your patient is seeing a therapist and is getting much worse, you need to be aware of it and you need to tactfully raise this concern with the patient and the therapist. This is both to ensure that the patient is being treated appropriately psychotherapeutically and to manage medico-legal liability. If there are negative events that occur in psychotherapy that result in a patient's self-harm behaviours, or suicide, a primary care provider is likely to be included in any litigation taken by the family.

The role of psychiatrists

When treating patients with personality disorders it is always best if psychiatrists can be involved in the care, either to manage the comorbid Axis I diagnosis or to facilitate some psychotherapeutic involvement. However, patients with personality disorders have been estimated to occur in five to 10 per cent of the population (Frances, 2005). Primary care providers are familiar with the difficulties in getting patients seen by psychiatrists who are not able to treat a large number of patients because of the labour-intensive nature of psychiatric care and other considerations.

Managing the clinician's reactions to the patient

Countertransference

It is important for primary care providers, even those who do not see themselves as psychotherapeutically oriented, to have some awareness of the concept of countertransference. Strictly speaking, countertransference is defined as the reaction the clinician has to the patient that mirrors significant past conflicts experienced by the clinician. However, a more useful and pragmatic definition of countertransference is to consider all reactions that patients evoke in clinicians. It is important for clinicians to be mindful of the reactions that patients evoke.

Sometimes the first diagnostic signal that there is a personality disorder component present in a patient is when the clinician looks at his or her schedule and sees the patient's name and says, "Oh no, not again, so soon." This should be a signal to the clinician to review whether or not there is some personality disorder component in the patient that has been overlooked.

The patient with a personality disorder can be seen as someone who by virtue of their temperament and their difficulties commonly induces negative feelings in the therapist. Understanding the feelings induced helps the clinician to understand the patient's dynamics. Also, being aware of the feelings induced allows clinicians to avoid the treatment mistakes that can occur when these feelings are not recognized. When clinicians meet people who feel "short-changed" by life, countertransference or counter-reactions naturally ensue.

If the clinician's own reactions are not well understood and/or recognized, there is a risk that medication will be either under-utilized (by not diagnosing the comorbid Axis I diagnosis), or over-utilized (to quell behaviours clinicians find disturbing). As well, countertransference can affect whether or not patients are seen regularly, too infrequently or too frequently. It is important to remember that these patients can elicit our rescue fantasies and we may see them more frequently than we are comfortable with, or conversely too infrequently for them. The correct frequency of seeing these patients is sometimes not as often as they may wish and not as infrequently as the clinician may wish.

It is also important to remember that if irritation with patients with personality disorders is not recognized, it will subtly colour the clinician's reactions (i.e., the tone in which comments are made). Some patients will respond to slight modulations in tone, or hesitations in responding to comments, by over-reacting and disrupting treatment. Other patients who come to feel that the clinician has passed the different tests that they have set for them will never want to leave treatment with that clinician and may develop dependency on the clinician, which poses its own counter-reactions.

Boundary violations

Unrecognized reactions that clinicians have to patients may cause boundary violations. There is a continuum of boundary violations from excess sessions, excess medications and favours (i.e., writing letters of support that are not consistent with the actual clinical facts), all the way to sexual boundary violations. Patients with personality disorders, because of their complicated histories and needs, are over-represented among those patients who become involved with their health care professionals.

There are different psychodynamics that such involvements may reflect. However, the crucial point for primary care providers is to maintain strict boundaries. The responsibility for boundary maintenance rests with the clinician. If clinicians find themselves doing things that they do not do for other patients, this is an early sign that there are boundary issues that require attention. Gutheil (Gutheil & Alexander, 1992) has pointed out that it is best to see one's self as a "coach," that is, stay on the sidelines and do not get in the game (i.e., avoid any type of engagement that constitutes a boundary violation).

Self-harm behaviours and suicide

Patients with borderline personality disorder may attempt to harm themselves at some point in their lives. The literature suggests that about 75 per cent will make a suicide attempt at some point and nine percent will complete suicide (Frances, 2005). Most primary care providers are familiar with how to assess and respond to acute suicidal risk (see also, "Assessment and management of suicide risk," page 237). A more particular challenge with these patients is that they are frequently chronically suicidal. The chronically suicidal patient may not be an acute risk. However, it is important to have a practical means of responding clinically to these patients and discharging the medico-legal liability so that safety is ensured.

With chronically suicidal patients it is important to convincingly convey to them that the clinician cannot take responsibility for their lives and that finding out if the clinician or anyone else cares cannot be learned by finding out what the clinician will do when patients try to harm themselves. It is helpful to clarify for patients that self-harm behaviour means that the treatment is not working and that the therapy may need to be reviewed.

Importance of ongoing assessment and documentation

Because patients with a personality disorder may harm themselves when they are overwhelmed, it is important to keep in mind the central importance of assessing and documenting risk (see also, "Assessment and management of suicide risk," page 237). Primary care providers should document self-harm assessment in all patients on all visits to manage and respond to this issue optimally and to demonstrate for medico-legal reasons that this has been done. Documentation should include that the patient currently does not demonstrate any self-harm (SH) ideation (I) or intent (I) today (T)—the mnemonic is "no SHIIT."

For the chronically suicidal patient it may be necessary to have a protocol for a continuum of assessment and documentation. The continuum of assessment and documentation includes:

· indicating that the patient is not actively suicidal at this time but remains a chronic risk dependent on future substance use, disappointment or stress
· reviewing and documenting what patients will do if they become actively suicidal (i.e., call a family member, call a crisis line, go to the nearest emergency room)
· discussing the treatment with a colleague to make sure that there is no medication or therapy approach that needs to be modified, as well as to note that the clinician has had this consultation
· noting that the colleague has agreed with the treatment is important in medico-legal risk management.

Conclusion

Primary care providers are on the front line in treating patients with difficult personality disorders. Recent research indicates better outcomes than previously assumed. A careful consideration of key assessment and treatment issues can help optimize outcome. This results in less pain for patients and their families (and their caregivers!).

References

American Psychiatric Association. (2001). *Practice Guideline for the Treatment of Patients with Borderline Personality Disorder*. Arlington, VA: Author.

American Psychiatric Association. (2000). *Diagnostic and Statistical Manual of Mental Disorders* (pp. 629–675). Washington, DC: Author.

Baldessarini, R.J., Tondo,L. & Davis, P. (2006). Decreased risk of suicides and attempts during long-term lithium treatment: A meta-analytic review. *Bipolar Disorders, 8*, 625–639.

Cipriani, A., Pretty, H., Hawton, K. & Geddes, J.R. (2005). Lithium in the prevention of suicidal behavior and all-cause mortality in patients with mood disorders: A systematic review of randomized trials. *American Journal of Psychiatry, 162*, 1805–1819.

Cowdry, R.W. (1992). Psychobiology and psychopharmacology of Borderline Personality Disorder. In D. Silver & M.B. Rosenbluth (Eds.), *Handbook of Borderline Disorders* (pp. 495–509). Madison, CT: International Universities Press, Inc.

Frances, A. (2005). Personality disorders. In K.R.R. Krishnan (Ed.), *Educational Review Manual in Psychiatry* (pp.1–34). New York: Castle Connolly Graduate Medical Publishing.

Gunderson, J.G., Weinberg, I., Daversa, M., Kueppenbender, K.D., Zanarini,M.C., Shea, T. et al. (2006). Descriptive longitudinal observations on the relationship of Borderline Personality Disorder and Bipolar Disorder. *American Journal of Psychiatry, 163*, 1173–1178.

Gutheil, T.G. & Alexander, V. (1992). Medicolegal issues between the Borderline patient and the therapist. In D. Silver & M.B. Rosenbluth (Eds.), *Handbook of Borderline Disorders* (pp. 335–389). Madison, CT: International Universities Press, Inc.

Kool. S., Schoevers, R., de Maat, S., Van, R., Molenaar,P., Vink, A. et al. (2005). Efficacy of pharmacotherapy in depressed patients with and without personality disorders: A systematic review and meta-analysis. *Journal of Affective Disorders, 88* (3), 269–278.

Linehan, M.M. (1992). Behaviour therapy, dialectics and the treatment of Borderline Personality Disorder. In D. Silver & M.B. Rosenbluth (Eds.), *Handbook of Borderline Disorders* (pp. 389–415). Madison, CT: International Universities Press, Inc.

Mulder, R.T. (2002). Personality pathology and treatment outcome in Major Depression: A review. *American Journal of Psychiatry, 159*, 359–371.

Zanarini, M.C., Frankenburg, F.R., Dubo, E.D., Sichel, A.E., Trikha, A., Levin, A. et al. (1998). Axis I comorbidity of Borderline Personality Disorder. *American Journal of Psychiatry, 155*, 1733–1739.

Zanarini, M.C., Frankenburg, F.R., Hennen, J., Reich, D.B. & Silk, K. (2004). Axis I comorbidity in patients with Borderline Personality Disorder: 6-year follow-up and prediction of time to remission. *American Journal of Psychiatry, 161*, 2108–2114.

10

The patient with dementia

KENNETH LE CLAIR AND DALLAS SEITZ

Epidemiology of dementia in Canada

Dementia is very common and becoming more prevalent with time.

Dementia currently affects 420,000 Canadians; more than 700,000 will be affected by 2031.

Most dementias are associated with older ages:
· Prevalence of dementia in people over 65 years old is eight per cent:
  - 65–74 years old: 2.4 per cent
  - 75–84 years: 12 per cent
  - > 85 years: 35 per cent
· Prevalence in long-term care is more than 60 per cent
· Incidence of dementia in people over 65 years old is one to two per cent annually.

Total economic costs to the Canadian economy associated with dementia are as follows:
· Annual economic costs of dementia in Canada: $5.5 billion.
· Annual cost per individual: mild dementia, $9,451; severe dementia, $36,794.

Dementia is common, costly, and lowers the threshold for other chronic and acute illnesses to produce significant disability.

Detection, diagnosis and differential diagnosis of dementia

Who is at risk for dementia? Red flags in primary care practice

MEDICAL RED FLAGS CHECKLIST
· Advanced age
· History of cardiovascular risk factors (hypertension, dyslipidemia, history of smoking, obesity, physical inactivity, diabetes, atrial fibrillation)
· History of cardiovascular disease or cerebrovascular disease
· A family history of dementia
· History of delirium or new onset depression in late life
· History of head trauma or neurological illness (Parkinson's)

BEHAVIOURAL RED FLAGS CHECKLIST
· Recent motor vehicle accident in older adult
· Difficulties in taking medication
· Missing appointments
· Repetitive calling to the office
· Family concerns about memory loss
· Deferring answers to questions to family members or caregivers

The P.I.E.C.E.S. checklist

A helpful approach to determining the differential diagnosis of cognitive impairment/dementia is the P.I.E.C.E.S. checklist, which was developed in Ontario as a provincial training strategy to enhance the ability of long-term care facility staff to meet the care requirements of individuals with complex physical and cognitive/mental health needs with associated behavioural issues. P.I.E.C.E.S. stands for:
· **P**hysical
· **I**ntellectual
· **E**motional
· **C**apabilities

· Environment
· Social.

Cognitive impairment can be a result of physical (P) or medical cause, or another intellectual (I) and/or emotional (E) disorder. The cognitive impairment/disorder, in turn, can be affected positively or negatively by the match between the capabilities (C) of the person and the demands being put on the person along with the person's environmental (E) and social (S) context and life course.

Primary care providers should use the P.I.E.C.E.S. checklist to determine the diagnosis and differential diagnosis, as well as to identify any comorbid conditions that may be affecting the quality of life of the person with cognitive impairment and/or dementia.

Differential diagnosis of dementia/cognitive impairment

Physical: Think delirium
· Delirium is common in hospitalized elderly undergoing surgery or acute medical illness.
· Individuals with dementia are at high risk for developing dementia with delirium.
· Sudden onset of cognitive decline may be associated with changes in level of consciousness.
· Delirium may fluctuate over the course of the day or several days.
· It is critical to differentiate delirium from a dementia or a superimposed delirium on top of a dementia (one of the major vulnerability factors for delirium is cognitive impairment/dementia).

See Figure 10.1 for an algorithm to detect and determine the cause of delirium.

Figure 10.1 Algorithm for diagnosing delirium

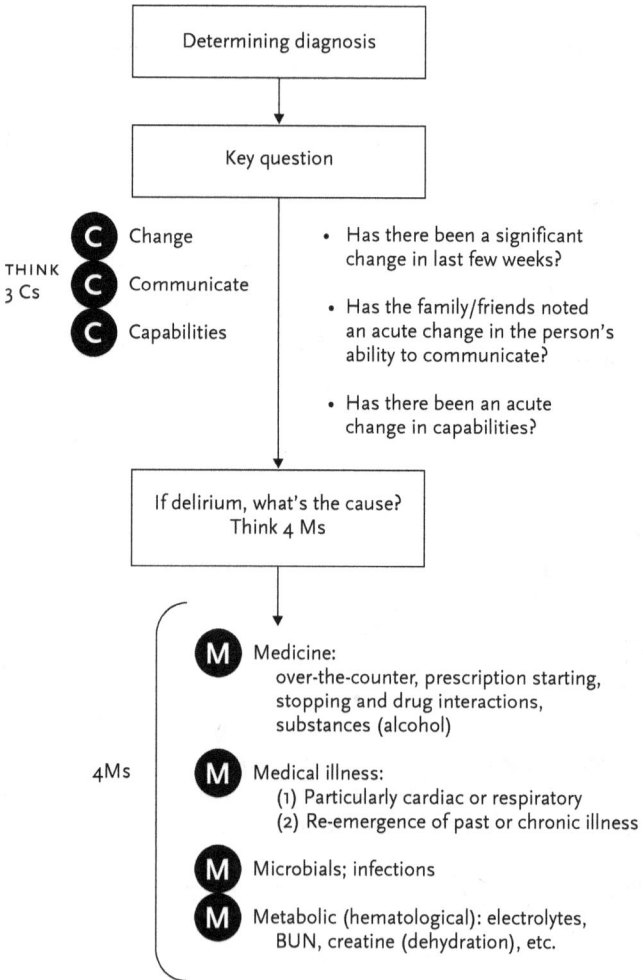

```
            ┌─────────────────────────┐
            │  Determining diagnosis  │
            └─────────────────────────┘
                         │
                         ▼
            ┌─────────────────────────┐
            │       Key question      │
            └─────────────────────────┘
                         │
```

(C) Change   • Has there been a significant
                          change in last few weeks?

THINK
3 Cs   **(C)** Communicate   • Has the family/friends noted
                                  an acute change in the person's
        (C) Capabilities   ability to communicate?

                                • Has there been an acute
                                  change in capabilities?

```
            ┌─────────────────────────────┐
            │ If delirium, what's the cause? │
            │        Think 4 Ms            │
            └─────────────────────────────┘
                         │
                         ▼
```

(M) Medicine:
        over-the-counter, prescription starting,
        stopping and drug interactions,
        substances (alcohol)

4Ms   **(M)** Medical illness:
                (1) Particularly cardiac or respiratory
                (2) Re-emergence of past or chronic illness

        (M) Microbials; infections

        (M) Metabolic (hematological): electrolytes,
                BUN, creatine (dehydration), etc.

Intellectual: Think normal aging and mild cognitive impairment

There are several other conditions to consider in the differential diagnosis of dementia in older adults.

NORMAL COGNITIVE CHANGES WITH AGE
- Aging typically involves slowing of cognitive processes with normal cognitive testing and no functional impairment.

MILD COGNITIVE IMPAIRMENT (MCI)
- MCI is an impairment in memory or other cognitive processes to an extent greater than that associated with normal aging.
- Cognitive testing shows decline (see "Montreal Cognitive Assessment (MoCA)" on page 170).
- The individual does not have functional impairment or dementia.
- There is a high risk for developing dementia. Of people with MCI, 13 per cent develop dementia per year.
- No treatments are currently available to prevent progression from MCI to dementia. Identify, monitor and treat risk factors and complete serial cognitive testing.

Emotional: Think depression or other psychiatric disorder

- Depression may present with cognitive changes, also known as "pseudodementia."
- Performance on cognitive testing varies. People often give "I don't know" answers rather than answering incorrectly.
- If depression is suspected, consider supportive tools such as the Geriatric Depression Scale and/or the Cornell Depression Scale.
- Late-life onset of depression may be associated with increased risk for subsequent dementia.

Table 10.1 Characteristic features of common types of dementia

	ALZHEIMER'S DEMENTIA	LEWY BODY DEMENTIA (LBD)	VASCULAR DEMENTIA	FRONTO-TEMPORAL DEMENTIA
Age at onset (average)	70–80	70–80	60–70	50–60
Percentage of dementia	50–60%	10–20%	10–20%	10% (higher proportion in ages < 60)
First symptoms	Short-term memory loss	Slowness, problems with visuospatial tasks	General slowing of cognition, may have depression at onset	Behavioural changes, language changes, apathy
Associated symptoms	Lack of insight into memory difficulties may be present early

History of mild cognitive impairment in some individuals

Co-occurring cerebrovascular disease common | Parkinsonian symptoms (rigidity, slowness, may not have tremor)

Hallucinations (often visual and non-frightening)

Early falls

Marked fluctuations in consciousness (can appear drowsy or delirious)

Sleep disturbance (REM sleep disorder – "act out" dreams) | Registration of events better than recall (more likely to recall when given cues)

"Patchy deficits": may have marked deficits in language with relative preservation in language

Pure vascular dementia less common than mixed vascular and AD | Eating disturbances, (overeating, carbohydrate craving)

Disinhibition

Loss of insight

Impairment in social skills

May be associated with movement disorders or motor neuron disease |

Family history	Increased risk of AD	Often no family history	Cardiovascular, cerebrovascular disease	Strong family history in many cases (20−40%)
Neurological signs	Absent early on	Parkinsonian symptoms	Many have focal weakness, reflex changes	Frontal release signs (grasp, glabellar tap, snout reflexes)
Progression	5−15 year course Slowly progressive 2−3 point decline yearly on MMSE	Rapid progression from onset to severe symptoms over few years	Variable "step-wise decline"	Rapidly progressive over few years

Differentiating the types of dementia

Although there are many pathophysiological processes that lead to dementia in older adults, distinguishing between different dementias can be challenging but important. In considering the differential diagnosis of dementia, distinguishing among several features may be helpful (see Table 10.1 on page 166 for characteristic features of common types of dementia). These features may help to determine the cause of the dementia while informing prognosis and management.

Common types of dementias

ALZHEIMER'S DEMENTIA

· Most common dementia, accounting for 50 to 60 per cent of all cases
· Characteristic gradual onset with progressive decline

DEMENTIA WITH LEWY BODIES
· Second most common type of dementia
· Associated with visual hallucinations, Parkinsonian motor symptoms, marked fluctuation in cognition or level of consciousness, sensitivity to extrapyramidal side-effects of antipsychotic medication

VASCULAR COGNITIVE IMPAIRMENT AND VASCULAR DEMENTIA
· May be caused by a single large stroke or accumulation of multiple subcortical strokes
· Often associated with Alzheimer's dementia (mixed dementia)
· 30 per cent of people with a stroke progress to dementia

FRONTOTEMPORAL DEMENTIA
· Early loss of social skills, disinhibited behaviours, apathy, and loss of insight
· Often has earlier onset than other dementias and is frequently associated with family history of frontotemporal dementia

How do I evaluate someone for cognitive impairment and/or dementia?

Included are some office-based assessments of cognitive function, as well as guidelines for laboratory testing and neuroimaging. All patients suspected of having dementia should have a recent physical examination, including a screening neurological examination and review of medications as a part of the evaluation.

Quick cognitive screening tests

Recommended here is a combination of screening tests that are feasible and that provide the ability to probe a number of brain functions, while also allowing the identification of early changes and changes over time.

This section describes a standard screening test, the Mini-Mental State Examination (MMSE), and a brief screening test called the Mini-Cog, followed by other recommended standardized tests.

MINI-MENTAL STATE EXAMINATION
The Mini-Mental State Examination (Folstein et al., 1975) is an 11-item test that takes five to 10 minutes to administer.
· Scoring: suggested cut-off score of 24 or less out of 30 should raise concerns regarding possible dementia
· Influenced by age, education
· Test items most sensitive to detection of dementia: orientation to date (especially year), delayed word recall, intersecting pentagons
· Pros: familiar; relatively short time to administer
· Cons: takes longer than other similar tests; tests limited number of cognitive domains (relatively less emphasis on memory and executive functioning); often not sensitive to early cognitive change

MINI-COG
The Mini-Cog (Borson et al., 2000) combines the delayed three-word recall and the clock-drawing test.

Test administration:
· First give the three-word registration: "I am going to say three words. I want you to repeat them back to me." Tell the patient that he or she will also be asked to recall them later.
· Then use the clock-drawing test (see below) as a distracter for the three-word recall. The scoring of the clock is similar to the Mini-Cog scoring described below.
· Then ask the patient to recall the three words.

Clock-drawing test
· One item, variations reported, one to two minutes to administer
· Test: "Please draw a clock and make the time show 10 minutes past 11:00"
· Scoring: normal (perfect or near perfect) or abnormal by inspection; any abnormal clock should raise suspicion for dementia and prompt further evaluation
· Pros: not influenced by age or education; easy, very quick and acceptable to most patients; some measure of visuospatial and executive function

· Cons: does not test memory or language abilities
· Recommended here for detecting and monitoring, including delirium

Scoring the Mini-Cog

The suggested scoring of the Mini-Cog is:
· three out of three on delayed recall indicates normal; zero out of three
  indicates likely dementia
· for one or two out of three on word recall: clock-drawing test normal =
  no dementia; clock-drawing test abnormal = dementia.

The Mini-Cog should be considered as a first-line cognitive screen in primary
care. Note that the Mini-Cog has not been evaluated as extensively as the
MMSE or the Montreal Cognitive Assessment (see below).

ANIMAL NAMING
· This is a word-generation test. Ask patients to name as many four-legged
  animals as they can in one minute.
· Tell patients that the test is not a race and that they will have one minute
  to complete the test from the point that they say the first word.
· People with dementia are 25 times more likely to name less than 10 animals
  in one minute.

MONTREAL COGNITIVE ASSESSMENT (MOCA)
The MoCA (available at www.mocatest.org; Nasreddine, et al., 2005)
is an 11-item test that takes 10 to 15 minutes to administer.
· Scoring: total score possible is 30 (like MMSE); 26 – 30 = likely normal;
  20 – 25 = possibly mild cognitive impairment or early dementia; < 20/30 =
  suspicious for dementia
· Good follow-up test if abnormalities are found on the clock-drawing test
  or Mini-Cog to further evaluate cognition or in individuals with cognitive
  complaints and normal scores on brief screening exams
· Test packages and instructions available online in multiple languages;
  adjustment for education is included in the testing (www.mocatest.org)

- Pros: free, easy to access and available in more than 20 languages; sensitive for dementia and mild cognitive impairment; tests executive function in detail and features a more rigorous memory section; trail-making section for evaluating for driving safety; very useful in primary care
- Cons: more time consuming than alternative tests; may be frustrating for those with more advanced cognitive impairment

Laboratory screening tests

Routine laboratory tests should include:
- complete blood count
- serum electrolytes
- serum calcium
- TSH and glucose.

Further investigations that may be useful in evaluating for possible dementia include measures of renal function and liver enzymes, and an ECG.

Indications for neuroimaging

Neuroimaging is not routinely recommended in the evaluation of dementia. Specific situations for which neuroimaging (CT scan of the head) should be considered include:
- age at dementia onset < 60
- focal neurological signs
- rapid progression of dementia
- recent head trauma
- use of anticoagulants
- unusual symptoms or gait disturbance.

Neuroimaging is also recommended to evaluate for concomitant cerebrovascular disease as this may affect subsequent management.

Assessing for dementia and/or cognitive impairment in the real world

Dementia and comorbid disorders

People in later age are most vulnerable for dementia. The prevalence of dementia, as noted previously, increases significantly among those over 65 years of age. The older the person, the higher the prevalence of dementia and comorbid disorders.

Patients who are older often have multiple chronic illnesses. Among people over age 65 in primary care, 80 per cent have at least one chronic illness and over 45 per cent have two or more. Also, many patients over age 65 have functional changes and disabilities associated with their multiple chronic disorders.

Patients in primary care with a possible dementia require a systematic, feasible approach that will:
· define the risks (e.g., roaming, driving, etc.; see page 173)
· provide a means of understanding and identifying the multiple causes
· set out a care plan that will address dementia and comorbid complexity
· enable the primary care provider to work effectively with the person, the family and the health care team.

A systematic but feasible approach has been developed in the P.I.E.C.E.S. program. The clinical foundation framework used in this program is the three-question template (3-Q template), which is an excellent framework for assessing an individual with dementia with comorbid conditions. For further information on the P.I.E.C.E.S. program and the three-question template, see the P.I.E.C.E.S. website (www.piecescanada.com).

The P.I.E.C.E.S three-question template

The three-question template is based on the following questions:
· What has changed? Think P.I.E.C.E.S. (physical, intellectual, emotional, capabilities, environment, social).

· What are the risks and causes (think P.I.E.C.E.S.)?
· What is the action (intervention, interaction and information)?

1. WHAT HAS CHANGED?

By asking this question "what has changed?" the primary care provider will gain insights into the diagnosis.

Defining what the person was able to do through his or her life that required cognitive abilities, and looking for changes in these abilities, will flag a possible dementia. This approach is much more sensitive than asking if a person does or does not possess an ability. This is because it is the "changes" that are critical red flags to possible cognitive impairment. The approach is also more effective than defining the chief complaint, as the chief complaint may only be what has been there for some time.

Identifying the changes also helps with the differential diagnosis. When a change occurs acutely, a clinician needs to think about delirium. An intermediate change that is predated by mood symptoms may point to a depression. Progressive, vague-onset change would suggest a dementia of the Alzheimer's type.

2. WHAT ARE THE "RISKS" AND CAUSES?

In patients with dementia it is critical to determine immediate risks and potential future risks. The acronym RISKS will give the primary care provider an opportunity to explore the breadth of common risks in people with cognitive impairment. These risks include:
· **R**oaming. Patients are prone to wandering. Identifying the degree to which wandering may put the person at risk for harm is critical.
· **I**mminent physical danger. This is particularly related to falls and fire.
· **S**uicide.
· **K**inship risks. This includes risks to others as well as possible elder abuse.
· **S**ubstance misuse and safe driving.

Using the P.I.E.C.E.S. approach allows the primary care provider to consider the range of factors that may contribute to, be the cause of, or influence the person with cognitive impairment.

The P.I.E.C.E.S. approach looks at the following factors:
· Physical: diseases, drugs, discomfort
· Intellectual: dementia, MCI
· Emotional: depression, psychosis
· Capabilities: activities of daily living (ADLs)
· Environment: over/understimulation, relocation, change in routine
· Social: care.

3. WHAT IS THE ACTION?
Primary care providers should think about "the three Is":
· What are the Investigations I need to do?
· What are the Interventions that I need to think about, both immediately and in the long term? This focuses particularly on the medical interventions.
· What are the Interactions that need to be considered? That is, what kind of psychosocial caregiver support do I need to think about and what do I need to discuss with the patient, family and colleagues? What information will enable effective response to treatment and/or flag critical factors for review and follow-up?

Management and critical issues in primary care

What medications can I use to treat dementia?

This section focuses on three groups of medications used in the management of Alzheimer's dementia (also see Table 10.2):
· the cholinesterase inhibitors
· the NMDA-receptor antagonist memantine
· medications used in treating risk factors, behaviour and mental health challenges associated with dementia.

CHOLINESTERASE INHIBITORS

In Canada, three cholinesterase inhibitors (also known as acetylcholinesterase inhibitors) are available:

- donepezil (Aricept)
- rivastigmine (Exelon)
- galantamine (Reminyl).

All three are currently approved for the treatment of mild to moderate Alzheimer's dementia. Donepezil is approved for severe Alzheimer's dementia. All have equal efficacy in the treatment of dementia.

Facts about cholinesterase inhibitors
- The target for cholinesterase inhibitors is to slow the rate of decline.
- All can cause similar side-effects.
- It is important to consider behavioural and functional outcomes in addition to cognitive scores in evaluating the effects of cholinesterase inhibitors
- Cholinesterase inhibitors may also be of benefit in vascular dementia, mixed vascular and Alzheimer's dementia, dementia with Lewy bodies, and dementia associated with Parkinson's disease.
- Cholinesterase inhibitors should not be used in frontotemporal dementia as they may worsen symptoms.

Clinical improvements noted with these medications:
- Modest improvements are noted in cognition and functioning with cholinesterase inhibitors.
- Most patients return to pretreatment baseline levels of dementia after six to 12 months of treatment.
- Most evidence is for the treatment of mild to moderate stages of dementia with emerging evidence to support the use of cholinesterase inhibitors in advanced stages of dementia.

MEMANTINE
- This newer medication targets NMDA receptors (glutamate) and reduces neurotoxicity accompanying Alzheimer's dementia.

- Most studies have evaluated the effects of memantine as an adjunct to treatment with cholinesterase inhibitors.
- Memantine is approved for treatment of moderate to severe dementia.
- It tends to be well tolerated. Typical side-effects may include confusion, dizziness and nausea.
- Dose adjustment is required in renal failure.
- Memantine is not covered under most public prescription plans.

OTHER MEDICATIONS
- ASA: not indicated for dementia but is used in treatment of comorbid cardiovascular or cerebrovascular disease
- Statins: no consistent evidence that they modify dementia risk in absence of other indications for their use
- Vitamin E: not recommended at present
- Estrogen: not recommended
- No natural products have been demonstrated to have effects on Alzheimer's dementia.

Health promotion and prevention of unnecessary disability
- Identify and treat cardiovascular risk factors and optimize cardiovascular health. This is critical not only in vascular dementia but also in Alzheimer's and other dementias.
- Encourage the patient to keep active in mind and body.
- Educate the patient and caregiver about early signs of delirium and common changes, including psychosis and depression.

Managing challenging behaviours associated with dementia
In addition to the cognitive changes of dementia, it is also common for people to develop behavioural and psychological symptoms of dementia (BPSD). BPSD is common, affecting between 40 and 80 per cent of people with dementia, and is associated with increased caregiver burden and increased likelihood of nursing home placement.

Table 10.2 Medications for the treatment of dementia

	DONEPEZIL (ARICEPT)	GALANTAMINE (REMINYL)	RIVASTIGMINE (EXELON)	MEMANTINE (EBIXA)
Initial dose*	5 mg	4 mg po bid (regular) 8 mg po od (extended release XR)	Oral: 1.5 mg po bid Patch: One 5 cm2 patch daily	5 mg po od
Titration schedule	Increase by 5 mg every 4 weeks	Increase by 8 mg every 4 weeks	Increase by 3 mg in divided doses every 4 weeks. Patch: Increase to one 10 cm2 patch daily after 4 weeks	Increase by 5 mg every week, start by adding second 5 mg dose
Maximum dose	10 mg	12 mg po bid 24 mg po od	6 mg po bid	10 mg po bid
Formulations	Tablets	Immediate release tablets taken bid, extended release tablet taken once daily	Tablet taken bid Transdermal patch recently released which is applied daily	Tablets given bid
Indications	Mild to moderate Alzheimer's disease	Mild to moderate Alzheimer's disease	Mild to moderate Alzheimer's disease	Adjunctive treatment added to cholinesterase inhibitor therapy in moderate to severe Alzheimer's disease

Table 10.2 Medications for dementia, continued

	DONEPEZIL (ARICEPT)	GALAN-TAMINE (REMINYL)	RIVASTIG-MINE (EXELON)	MEMANTINE (EBIXA)
Other potential indications	Vascular dementia Emerging evidence in severe dementia	Evidence in mixed Alzheimer's and vascular dementia	Best supported treatment in Parkinson's dementia and dementia with Lewy bodies	
Side-effects	Contraindicated with history of sick-sinus syndrome, left bundle branch block, recent peptic ulcer disease Common side-effects: Muscle cramps Insomnia Nausea Diarrhea (MIND)	Similar to donepezil	Similar to donepezil Gastro-intestinal side-effects often more pronounced	Common side-effects: Confusion Headache Equilibrium (dizziness) Constipation Kidney (requires dose adjustment in renal failure as per CPS) (CHECK)
Other notes				At publication, not covered on any provincial drug formularies; cost is ~$200.00/month

*All cholinesterase inhibitors should be given in the morning to minimize sleep disturbance. Lower starting doses and slower dose titration may be necessary in some individuals who are sensitive to side-effects.

BPSD can emerge at any stage of dementia and can include behaviours such as:
· agitation and restlessness
· anxiety
· apathy/failure to participate; withdrawing/crying
· defensive behaviour
· hearing and seeing things that do not exist
· hoarding and/or rummaging
· impulsivity
· inappropriate sexual behaviour
· intrusiveness
· resistance to care
· suspicious/accusing others
· vocally disruptive behaviour
· wandering.

WHAT STEPS SHOULD I TAKE IN EVALUATING AND TREATING THESE
BEHAVIOURS?

Obtain a clear description of the behaviour using the ABC approach:
· What are the *Antecedents* to the behaviour?
· What exactly is the *Behaviour*? (Be more specific than "agitated" or "aggressive.")
· What is the *Consequence* (caregiver's response) of the behaviour?

After obtaining a clear description, the next step should be to rule out
potential reversible secondary causes of the behaviour. Evaluate delirium
risk using the three-question template on page 172 (what has changed? what
are the risks and causes? what is the action?) to enable a systematic
and comprehensive approach. Delirium can present with behavioural
disturbances in older adults with dementia and should first be ruled out
(see the algorithm for diagnosing delirium in Figure 10.1 on page 164).
Also, potential medical conditions that may exacerbate behaviours include
pain, unmet needs, constipation or environmental contributors.

Initiate non-pharmacological management for the specific behaviours. Provide education to caregivers, which can often decrease distress and negative responses to behaviours. Pharmacological treatments may need to be considered early if the behaviours are endangering others or cause extreme distress.

To determine the impact of the behaviour and the risks associated with the behaviour, and to monitor response, use the four Ds approach:
· Is the behaviour *Dangerous, Distressing, Disturbing* relationships or jeopardizing independence due to the effects on the caregivers, and/or causing *Disability* (i.e., medical malnutrition, risk for falls)?

If the behaviour persists, consider optimizing the treatment of the underlying dementia. This may include the appropriate use of preventative measures to prevent further cognitive decline along with prescription of cognitive enhancers if appropriate.

Evaluate and treat possible co-existing depression or anxiety using appropriate pharmacotherapy (e.g., SSRIs) and psychosocial interventions.

If these interventions fail, next consider pharmacotherapy directed at the behavioural and psychological symptoms of dementia (BPSD). Consider referral to psychiatry, neurology or geriatric medicine.

ARE THERE ANY MEDICATIONS THAT CAN BE USED IN TREATING BPSD?
In addition to treating the underlying dementia with appropriate psychosocial and pharmacological treatment, there are several medications that have demonstrated efficacy in treating certain BPSD behaviours (see Table 10.3 on page 181).

Behaviours that generally are not amenable to pharmacotherapy include wandering, repetitive questioning or vocalizing, abnormal eating behaviours, perseverative behaviours, inappropriate dressing or undressing, inappropriate defecation or urination.

Table 10.3 Medications for treatment of behavioural and psychological symptoms of dementia

RISPERIDONE	OLANZA-PINE	QUETIA-PINE	CITALO-PRAM	TRAZO-DONE
Indications				
Atypical antipsychotics are best supported treatment for BPSD			Similar to antipsychotics Second-line treatment for severe aggression or agitation (start with atypical)	Sleep disturbance associated with dementia Treatment of behaviours in fronto-temporal dementia
Initial dose				
0.25 od or bid	2.5 mg po qhs	12.5−25 mg po bid or qhs	10 mg	25 mg po qhs
Titration schedule				
Increase by 0.25−0.5 mg every 2−4 weeks	Increase by 2.5 mg every 2−4 weeks	Increase by 25−50 mg every 2−4 weeks	10 mg every 2−4 weeks	25 mg every 2−4 weeks
Maximum dose				
2 mg	10 mg	200 mg	40 mg	150 mg

Table 10.3 Medications for dementia, continued

Side-effects

RISPERIDONE	OLANZA-PINE	QUETIA-PINE	CITALO-PRAM	TRAZO-DONE
All antipsychotics can cause: sedation, falls, orthostatic hypotension, weight gain, impaired glucose tolerance, dyslipidemia			All SSRIs can cause: Headache Anorexia Nausea Diarrhea Sleep problems (HANDS) Increased risk of bleeding. Monitor for hyponatremia	Highly sedating Orthostatic hypotension Rarely may cause priapism

Monitoring

RISPERIDONE	OLANZA-PINE	QUETIA-PINE	CITALO-PRAM	TRAZO-DONE
Fasting lipids and glucose, gait, extrapyramdidal symptoms			Serum sodium, hemoglobin	

Special notes

RISPERIDONE	OLANZA-PINE	QUETIA-PINE	CITALO-PRAM	TRAZO-DONE
Most likely to cause EPS, especially at higher doses. Increased risk of mortality and possibly stroke with all atypical antipsychotics*	Most likely to cause weight gain and metabolic side-effects. Less EPS than risperidone. More sedating than risperidone	Very sedating Least likely to cause EPS, should be used first in Parkinson's and Lewy body dementia	Emerging evidence suggests it may be as effective as antipsychotics. Also effective in treating behaviours associated with frontotemporal dementia	Usually in treatment of sleep disturbance associated with dementia

* All atypical antipsychotics (risperidone, olanzapine, quetiapine) are associated with an increased risk of mortality in older adults with dementia. This increased risk in studies was approximately one per cent greater than that observed with placebo. Similar increased risk of stroke in older adults with dementia treated with antipsychotics.

Behaviours that may be responsive to pharmacological therapy include:
- verbal aggression
- anxiety
- agitation
- sadness
- insomnia
- sleep disturbances
- hyperactivity
- persistent delusions or hallucinations
- sexually inappropriate behaviour accompanied by agitation.

Atypical antipsychotics
Atypical antipsychotics are the best supported treatment for severe agitation or psychosis in dementia that is unresponsive to non-pharmacological interventions. The potential benefits of these medications must be balanced with potential serious adverse effects. Atypical antipsychotics have been associated with an increased risk of death and stroke when used to treat BPSD. Patients need to be warned of the potential risks of therapy and monitored carefully for adverse events.

Other medications
Other medications with some evidence for use in BPSD include SSRIs (e.g., citalopram) and the antidepressant trazodone. There is little or no evidence to support the use of benzodiazepines or other hypnotics. In addition, as there are significant safety concerns associated with their use, they are not recommended.

GENERAL PRINCIPLES OF USING PHARMACOTHERAPY IN DEMENTIA
When treating a patient with dementia with pharmacotherapy:
- start low and go slow
- use one medication at a time

· use medications at optimal dose and duration prior to switching or discontinuing
· use medications that will not worsen cognition
· be aware for drug–drug interactions.

Also, as dementia progresses, certain behaviours may no longer be problematic and medications may be discontinued gradually after several consecutive months of behavioural stability.

Beyond cognition: Five critical areas to assess in dementia

Assess the caregiver

While collateral information from the caregiver is essential in the assessment of dementia, be sure to assess for caregiver stress and implement strategies to decrease caregiver stress, including:
· enlisting additional supports, both informal and formal, through referral to home care agencies
· assisting in managing challenging behaviours
· discussing the role of respite care
· identifying and treating caregiver depression
· providing psychoeducation and directing to self-help and psychoeducational materials such as *The 36-Hour Day* (see the references at the end of this chapter).

Assess functional abilities

Any change in functional abilities in older adults should trigger an evaluation for dementia.

Assessing functional abilities is emphasized here because dementia and comorbid medical conditions may have an impact on functioning. The levels of support necessary to care for the individual in the community will depend on how these affect self-care.

Obtain caregiver and patient report of any change in activities of daily living. Instrumental activities (see below) are impaired before basic activities of daily living.

Review changes in basic activities of daily living (ADL):
· ambulation
· bathing
· continence
· dressing
· eating
· toileting
· transfers.

Review changes in instrumental activities of daily living (IADL):
· shopping
· household maintenance
· finance management
· meal preparation
· telephone use (especially knowledge of emergency contacts)
· transportation
· medication management.

Assess driving
Cessation of driving is inevitable for all older adults with progressive dementia. Discussions of driving cessation should begin early in the course of illness.

For those individuals with early dementia, discuss strategies to reduce risk of accidents (i.e., limit driving to familiar environments, drive while supervised, drive only in the daytime, minimize distractions in vehicle).

Moderate to severe dementia is a contraindication to driving. Moderate dementia is the loss of two or more instrumental activities of daily living. Severe dementia indicates inability to perform one or more of the basic activities of daily living.

Canadian guidelines suggest that cognitive impairment associated with loss of ability to complete two instrumental activities of daily living means that the individual is likely unfit to continue driving.

Review the Canadian Medical Association's publication *Determining Medical Fitness to Operate Motor Vehicles* (www.cma.ca/index.cfm/ci_id/18223/la_id/1.htm).

In general:
· Consider medical problems and medications that may elevate the risk for unsafe driving.
· Be familiar with your province's requirements for reporting fitness to drive.
· Beyond dementia, assess other critical factors required for driving (i.e., mobility, vision, emotional stability, other medical conditions).

REVIEW BY HISTORY
Ask the patient about:
· any recent accidents or near misses
· any incidents of becoming disoriented or lost while driving
· previous driving habits.

Assess capacity for treatment, finances and personal care

Capacity refers to a person's ability to *understand* information regarding decisions and their ability to *appreciate* how that information applies to their situation. Capacity is task- and situation-specific. Incapacity in one area does not necessarily mean that the individual is incapable in all areas of decision making.

There are several areas that are important to assess:
· treatment decisions
· consent to long-term care
· testamentary capacity (ability to complete a will)
· capacity to assign a power of attorney.

Assess future planning

In the context of a diagnosis of dementia, if the patient is capable, discuss matters such as:

· writing wills
· making advanced directives
· assigning powers of attorney for care and finances.

Involve the family in discussions about the course of dementia and long-term care planning.

When should I consider referral for further evaluation?

Primary care providers should consider referring the patient when there is:
· uncertainty over diagnosis after initial evaluation and treatment
· an indication for neuropsychological testing to differentiate between normal aging and mild cognitive impairment
· significant depression with poor response to treatment
· difficulties in tolerating medications for dementia
· challenging behaviours or significant stress on the caregiver and social environment
· need for genetic counselling
· patient or family request
· an indication for further evaluation of in-home safety, driving or other areas of potential risk.

What referrals should I consider to help support my patient with dementia?

· Alzheimer Society's First Link program for those newly diagnosed with dementia
· Home care services (e.g., in Ontario contact the local Community Care Access Centre)
· Psychiatry/neurology
· Geriatric medicine

Community and online resources

· Canadian Coalition for Seniors Mental Health (www.ccsmh.ca). Contains tools, evidence-based guidelines including guidelines on management of psychiatric problems in long-term care (focused on dementia), delirium, depression and suicide. All guidelines are free to download.

· Alzheimer Society of Canada (www.alzheimer.ca). Provides information for patients, families and clinicians on recent developments in dementia research and local support groups. The website contains numerous links for families and patients with regional contact information for provincial Alzheimer Society offices, and online videos and documents for families and caregivers.

· Canadian Consensus Guidelines on the Diagnosis and Treatment of Dementia (www.cccdtd.ca). Provides free, comprehensive, Canadian guidelines on dementia, mild cognitive impairment and other issues related to aging and cognition.

· The Driving and Dementia Toolkit (www.rgpeo.com/en/resources/Dementia-Toolkit.pdf). A resource for use in primary care that includes information on evaluating driving in dementia and provides helpful screening questions and approaches to discussing driving safety with patients and families.

· CMA Driver's Guide: *Determining Medical Fitness to Operate Motor Vehicles* (www.cma.ca/index.cfm/ci_id/18223/la_id/1.htm). Contains the Canadian Medical Association's guidelines on the evaluation of driving in dementia.

· Dementia Guide (www.dementiaguide.com). Provides caregivers with an online resource that explains behaviours associated with dementia, and provides online tools to chart behaviours over time to evaluate interventions.

· P.I.E.C.E.S. (www.piecescanada.com). Provides further information on the P.I.E.C.E.S. approach including job aids for assessment and psychotropic use.

· American Medical Association's *Physician's Guide to Assessing and Counseling Older Drivers* (www.ama-assn.org/ama/pub/category/10791.html). A useful document for evaluating older drivers that presents information on evaluating driving safety, including assessment of cognition and physical status.

Acknowledgments

The authors would like to thank Dr. Bill Dalziel, Dr. Marie-France Rivard and the P.I.E.C.E.S. consultation team for allowing us to use tools and resources that they have developed to provide education to primary care physicians.

References

Borson, S., Scanlan, J., Brush, M., Vitaliano, P. & Dokmak, A. (2000). The Mini-Cog: A cognitive "vital signs" measure for dementia screening in multi-lingual elderly. *International Journal of Geriatric Psychiatry, 15* (11), 1021–1027. DOI: 10.1002/1099-1166(200011)15:11<1021::AID-GPS234>3.0.CO;2-6

Canadian Study of Health and Aging Working Group (1994). Canadian study of health and aging: Study methods and prevalence of dementia. *Canadian Medical Association Journal, 150* (6), 899–913.

Feldman, H.H., Jacova, C., Robillard, A., Garcia, A., Chow, T., Borrie, M. et al. (2008). Diagnosis and treatment of dementia: 2. Diagnosis. *Canadian Medical Association Journal, 178* (7), 825–836. DOI: 10.1503/cmaj.070798

Folstein, M.F., Folstein, S.E. & McHugh, P.R. (1975). "Mini-mental state." A practical method for grading the cognitive state of patients for the clinician. *Journal of Psychiatric Research, 12* (3), 189–198. DOI: 10.1016/0022-3956(75)90026-6

Holsinger, T., Deveau, J., Boustani, M. & Williams, J.W. (2007). Does this patient have dementia? *Journal of the American Medical Association, 297* (21), 2391–2404.

Mace, N.L. & Rabins, P.V. (2001). *The 36-Hour Day: A Family Guide to Caring for Persons with Alzheimer Disease, Related Dementing Illnesses, and Memory Loss in Later Life.* New York: Warner Books.

Nasreddine, Z.S., Phillips, N.A., Bédirian, V., Charbonneau, S., Whitehead, V., Collin, I. et al. (2005). The Montreal Cognitive Assessment, MoCA: A brief screening tool for Mild Cognitive Impairment. *Journal of the American Geriatrics Society.* 53 (4), 695–699.

Patterson, C., Feightner, J.W., Garcia, A., Hsiung, G.Y.R., MacKnight, C. & Sadovnick, A.D. (2008). Diagnosis and treatment of dementia: 1. Risk assessment and primary prevention of Alzheimer disease. *Canadian Medical Association Journal, 178* (5), 548–556. DOI: 10.1503/cmaj.070796

Patterson, C.J.S., Gauthier, S., Bergman, H., Cohen, C.A., Feightner, J.W., Feldman, H. et al. (1999). Canadian Consensus Conference on Dementia: A physician's guide to using the recommendations. *Canadian Medical Association Journal, 160* (12), 1738–1742.

Peterson, R.C., Doody, R., Kurz, A., Mohs, R.C., Morris, J.C., Rabins, P.V. et al. (2001). Current concepts in mild cognitive impairment. *Archives of Neurology, 58* (12), 1985–1992.

Sink, K.M., Holder, K.R. & Yaffe, K. (2005). Pharmacological treatment of neuropsychiatric symptoms of dementia: A review of the evidence. *Journal of the American Medical Association, 293* (5), 596–608.

11

The adult patient with ADHD

UMESH JAIN

Epidemiology of ADHD

Attention-deficit/hyperactivity disorder (ADHD) is the most common neurobiological disorder in childhood. At least 60 per cent of this population continues into adulthood with impairing symptoms, leading to a possible prevalence rate for ADHD of 4.4 per cent among adults.

By adulthood, almost as many females present with this condition as males. ADHD affects people in every socioeconomic group and is found in every country in the world, with some countries having higher prevalence rates than Canada.

Common questions about adult ADHD

How did 4.4 per cent of the population suddenly have ADHD?
Until 1994, there were no diagnostic criteria for adult ADHD so clinicians were forced to give another diagnosis to account for the clinical presentation.

What would it have been called if not ADHD?
The natural course of ADHD is to move toward anxiety and depression. Also consider ADHD in patients with Bipolar II disorder, personality disorders, concurrent addictions to cannabis and cocaine, and generalized anxiety disorder.

Won't ADHD patients abuse their medications?
To the contrary, the medications have a protective role in preventing the patient from self-medicating.

Isn't ADHD just an excuse for bad habits and a lazy attitude?
ADHD is highly treatable. Providing treatment when symptoms are present will give patients an opportunity to live to their potential.

Doesn't everyone have some ADHD?
Anyone can have some of the symptoms of ADHD, but to meet the criteria for the diagnosis a number of symptoms must be present and they must be causing significant impairment.

The patient only wants the medication now and then. Is that possible?
Yes, while the medications should be seen as facilitating the non-drug agenda, some patients only need medications in situations of high attentional load.

My patient is not hyperactive—could she still have ADHD?
We likely miss many of the patients who have only the inattentive symptoms of ADHD such as being shy or withdrawn, or being "daydreamers." As a general rule, patients who have only the inattentive symptoms are often female.

Isn't ADHD just a reflection of our Western lifestyle and the latest "fad" of the media?
ADHD is prevalent around the world and not just in Western countries. The existence of childhood ADHD has been well accepted for decades. Only since the late 1980s have outcome studies shown that the disorder continues into adulthood.

Common presentation of adults with ADHD
Where the core symptoms in childhood ADHD are inattention, impulse control problems and motor hyperactivity, impulse control problems and motor hyperactivity generally soften by adolescence, but inattention remains.

The associated symptoms of ADHD are equally problematic for patients though not diagnostic. The patient:

· procrastinates and has poor time-management skills
· has poor organizational skills
· feels rushed and/or misses the subtleties of information
· has problems in interpersonal relationships, including parenting skills
· appears to not take responsibility for himself or herself
· has difficulty delivering (e.g., missed deadlines)
· has difficulty paying bills, completing reports or assignments ("paper is kryptonite" to the person with ADHD).

The following should *not* be used to dismiss a diagnosis of ADHD

The following clinical observations are not sufficient to rule out a diagnosis of ADHD:*

· The clinician does not observe hyperactivity in the office.
· The patient reports a great deal of problems with organization, time management and executive function but is reliable in keeping appointments, filling out forms and paying for treatment.
· The patient comes in saying he or she has read about ADHD and thinks he or she has this problem.
· There is no family history.
· The spouse or parent suggests symptoms of ADHD, which the patient dismisses.
· The patient is well educated or employed in a high-level position.
· The patient is very bright, and early school report cards do not describe problems with attention or behaviour. For some, increased autonomy and challenge led to evidence of impairment in later years. Other patients may, on further exploration, give a very convincing account of unusual coping strategies such as excess time on homework or increased need for assistance.
· The patient was clearly hyperactive, impulsive and inattentive when younger but currently only has difficulty with a few residual symptoms. In some, impairment is still clinically significant.

· The patient does not remember or denies symptoms in childhood, and school report cards are not available. Usually a careful developmental history will reveal evidence of the impact of the disorder, even if the patient did not have insight, either at the time or presently, into the symptoms that provoked these consequences.

*Reproduced with permission from the Canadian Attention Deficit Hyperactivity Disorder Resource Alliance *Canadian ADHD Practice Guidelines*, 2nd Edition (Turgay et al., 2008).

How to screen for adult ADHD in five minutes (rapid assessment)

If patients have experienced any of the following high-yield situations, then ADHD *must* be considered:
· Their child or any first-degree family member was diagnosed with ADHD.
· They were diagnosed with ADHD as a child or adolescent.
· They felt a calming, focused sensation on a psychostimulant, cannabis or cocaine.
· They had psychometric testing as a child or adolescent suggesting they had a learning disability and particularly a problem of working memory.
· The patient or their loved one says, "I think I [they] have ADHD."
If the answer is "yes" to any of the above, then give the patient the Adult ADHD Self-Report Scale (Kessler et al., 2005), which is included as an appendix to the downloadable *Canadian ADHD Practice Guidelines* from the Canadian ADHD Resource Alliance (www.caddra.ca). This scale *does not make the diagnosis* and does not have a threshold marker, but the questionnaire will help determine if the adult ADHD diagnosis should be considered when most of the questions are answered in the affirmative.

Steps to consider if ADHD is suspected
· Apply the DSM criteria to the patient to determine if the patient has symptoms (see page 195).
· Use the assessment form (CADDRA Assessment Form #2 Adult) available as part of the *Canadian ADHD Practice Guidelines* (www.caddra.ca) to help take the history and guide the management. This is the recognized

Canadian standard and it can be photocopied or downloaded directly and put into the medical record.

- Use the Weiss Functional Impairment Rating Scale — Self-Report (WFIRS-S) to document a patient's baseline level of impairment, and use it sequentially to determine if the treatment is moving the patient to normal functioning.
- If a suspected learning disability is also in the differential diagnosis, consider a referral to a community psychologist. This is expensive but necessary when problems are arising in areas such as organizational problems (i.e., executive functioning deficits), reading comprehension (e.g., making mistakes in reading, particularly in work situations) and graphomotor problems (e.g., their handwriting can't keep up with how fast they are processing information).
- Begin the psychoeducational process (see page 197).

DSM-IV-TR Criteria for Attention-Deficit/Hyperactivity Disorder

A. Either (1) or (2):

(1) six (or more) of the following symptoms of **inattention** have persisted for at least 6 months to a degree that is maladaptive and inconsistent with developmental level:

Inattention

   (a) often fails to give close attention to details or makes careless mistakes in schoolwork, work, or other activities

   (b) often has difficulty sustaining attention in tasks or play activities

   (c) often does not seem to listen when spoken to directly

   (d) often does not follow through on instructions and fails to finish school work, chores, or duties in the workplace (not due to oppositional behavior or failure to understand instructions)

   (e) often has difficulty organizing tasks and activities

   (f) often avoids, dislikes, or is reluctant to engage in tasks that require sustained mental effort (such as schoolwork or homework)

(g) often loses things necessary for tasks or activities (e.g., toys, school assignments, pencils, books, or tools)

(h) is often easily distracted by extraneous stimuli

(i) is often forgetful in daily activities

(2) six (or more) of the following symptoms of **hyperactivity-impulsivity** have persisted for at least 6 months to a degree that is maladaptive and inconsistent with developmental level:

Hyperactivity

(a) often fidgets with hands or feet or squirms in seat

(b) often leaves seat in classroom or in other situations in which remaining seated is expected

(c) often runs about or climbs excessively in situations in which it is inappropriate (in adolescents or adults, may be limited to subjective feelings of restlessness)

(d) often has difficulty playing or engaging in leisure activities quietly

(e) is often "on the go" or often acts as if "driven by a motor"

(f) often talks excessively

Impulsivity

(g) often blurts out answers before questions have been completed

(h) often has difficulty awaiting turn

(i) often interrupts or intrudes on others (e.g., butts into conversations or games)

B. Some hyperactive-impulsive or inattentive symptoms that caused impairment were present before age 7 years.

C. Some impairment from the symptoms is present in two or more settings (e.g., at school [or work] and at home).

D. There must be clear evidence of clinically significant impairment in social, academic, or occupational functioning.

E. The symptoms do not occur exclusively during the course of a Pervasive
    Developmental Disorder, Schizophrenia, or other Psychotic Disorder and
    are not better accounted for by another mental disorder (e.g., Mood Disorder,
    Anxiety Disorder, Dissociative Disorders, or a Personality Disorder).

Code based on type:

314.01 Attention-Deficit/Hyperactivity Disorder, Combined Type: if both Criteria
A1 and A2 are met for the past 6 months

314.00 Attention-Deficit/Hyperactivity Disorder, Predominantly Inattentive Type:
if Criterion A1 is met but Criterion A2 is not met for the past 6 months

**314.01 Attention-Deficit/Hyperactivity Disorder, Predominantly Hyperactive-
Impulsive Type**: if Criterion A2 is met but Criterion A1 is not met for the past
6 months

Coding note: For individuals (especially adolescents and adults) who currently
have symptoms that no longer meet full criteria, "In Partial Remission" should
be specified.

Reprinted with permission from the *Diagnostic and Statistical Manual of Mental Disorders*,
Fourth Edition, Text Revision (Copyright 2000). American Psychiatric Association.

Treatment options

Psychoeducation is the first step to a treatment approach
· Evidence shows that even well-treated people with ADHD will deteriorate
  without changes to lifestyle.
· ADHD is highly impairing in many domains and the patient may want
  to rush the agenda by starting medications immediately. Resist the urge
  to initiate medications without adequately educating the patient.
· A patient who follows through on the agenda is also showing commitment
  to the process.
· There is much to know and knowledge is power. This reduces dependency
  on the clinician.

Medical treatment

See Table 11.1 on page 200 for details about medical treatment of adults for simple ADHD.

GENERAL PRINCIPLES

· Start with a very low dose. Increase the dose and stop when the target symptoms are better.
· Resist the urge to "see if a little more makes a difference."
· Use long-acting agents over short-acting ones as they produce better compliance and better effect.
· If another family member is being treated for ADHD, use the medication that the first family member has been successfully treated with as it will likely have a positive effect on the subsequent patient.
· Combining the medications for ADHD with antidepressants, mood stabilizers or other psychiatric medications is common. Review any potential drug interaction.
· Always ensure the patient is medically stable before medications are started as there are known risks to the patient that must be reviewed. Review the product monograph. All ADHD medications are known to have risk to the CV system in that they all increase blood pressure and increase heart rate. It is not necessary to do a pre-treatment ECG. However, some patients are at a higher risk and should be referred for assessment before treatment if they have any of the following:
  - a history of unresolved structural cardiac problems
  - a family history of known cardiac conduction problems
  - an unexplained syncope.

MEDICAL TREATMENT OF ADULTS FOR SIMPLE ADHD

· Treat the ADHD symptoms first and then see what remains. The exception might be in cases of suspected Bipolar I disorder where the mood stabilizer should come first.
· While long-acting agents are preferred, augmentation of short-acting psychostimulants could be used to account for variations in day-to-day attention loads.

· Do pre- and post-reviews of medication efficacy and side-effects. Use
  the Side-Effect Rating Scale in the *Canadian ADHD Practice Guidelines*
  (www.caddra.ca).
· Monitor patients on a bimonthly basis until they are at their correct dose
  and every three months thereafter.

Non-medical treatment
· **Behavioural interventions**: Lifestyle management is critical. Bad habits
  have to be changed. The role of the primary care clinician is to assist
  patients in finding resources to facilitate their lifestyle changes.
· **Occupational therapists**: Occupational therapists can be very useful
  in helping to create organizational plans and reviewing basic life skills.
· **ADHD coach**: While there are few trained coaches, they can help patients
  reach their goals.
· **Electronic strategies**: Reducing clutter and reorganizing information using
  computer-based technologies, PDAs and software can help in dealing with
  the "paper problems."
· **Vocational assessment**: This can assist the patient in workplace situations
  and help the person advocate for the required accommodations.
· **Community support networks**: ADHD support groups can support the
  psychological needs of the patient and identify strategies that others have
  found useful. Often, spouses get the most benefit as they develop a better
  understanding of their partners.

Psychological treatment
ADHD can lead to significant problems of low self-esteem, decreased self-
confidence and strife in interpersonal relationships. When the diagnosis of
ADHD is made, it can cause both relief as well as despair, as the person may
reflect on lost opportunities due to non-treatment when they were younger.
In any case, a psychological agenda is critical.

Table 11.1 Medical treatment for ADHD uncomplicated—adults

Alphabetically listed. Refer to product monographs for complete prescribing information

BRAND NAME (ACTIVE CHEMICAL)	DOSAGE FORM	START-ING DOSE	TITRATION SCHEDULE EVERY 7 DAYS		MAXIMUM DAILY (>70 KG)[1, 2]	
			As per product mono-graph	As per CAD-DRA board	As per product mono-graph	As per CAD-DRA board*
First-line agents – Long-acting preparations (includes off-label use)						
Adderall XR (amphet-amine mixed salts)	5, 10, 15, 20, 25, 30 mg cap	10 mg q.d. a.m	☐ 10 mg	☐ 10 mg	20–30 mg	50 mg
Biphentin (methylphe-nidate HCl)	10, 15, 20, 30, 40, 50, 60, 80 mg cap	10–20 mg q.d. a.m.	☐ 10 mg	☐ 10 mg	80 mg	80 mg[3]
Concerta (methylphe-nidate HCl)	18, 27, 36, 54 mg tab	18 mg q.d. a.m.	☐ 18 mg	☐ 18 mg	72 mg	108 mg
Strattera (atomox-etine)	10, 18, 25, 40, 60, 80, 100 mg cap	40 mg[4] q.d. for 7–14 days	Maintain dose for a min. of 7–14 days before adjust-ing to 60 then 80 mg/ day max. dose/day 1.4 mg/ kg/day or 100 mg[5]	Maintain dose for a min. of 7–14 days before adjusting. 60 then 80 mg/ day max dose/day 1.4 mg/kg/ day or 100 mg[5]	Lesser of 1.4 mg/ kg/day or 100 mg/day	Lesser of 1.4 mg/ kg/day or 100 mg/ day

Vyvanse (lisdexamfetamine dimesylate)	20, 30, 40, 50, 60 mg cap	20–30 mg q.d. a.m.	by clinical discretion	☐ 10 mg	60 mg	70 mg

* Doses per CADDRA Board that are over product monograph maximum doses should be considered off-label use. A consensus decision has been made based on clinical use and research data.

[1] Maximum off-label doses have been published in the AACAP Practice Parameters but the off-label maximums are either the same or lower in the CAP-G based on the CADDRA Board.

[2] The maximum daily dose can be split into once daily (q.d.), twice daily (b.i.d.) or three times daily (t.i.d.) doses except for once a day formulations.

[3] While the theoretical maximum off-label dose for Biphentin could be 100 mg, clinical practice currently suggests that 80 mg is the maximum that is used.

[4] Some adults may better tolerate a lower starting dose of 25 mg.

[5] Strattera titration schedule applies to children and adolescents over 70 kg body weight and adults.

Second-line or adjunctive agents – Short-acting and intermediate-acting stimulant preparations**

Dexedrine (dextro-amphet-amine sulphate)	5 mg tab	2.5–5 mg b.i.d.	☐ 5 mg	☐ 5 mg	40 mg	50 mg
Dexedrine Spansule[6] (dextro-amphetamine sulphate)	10, 15 mg cap	10 mg q.d. a.m.	☐ 5 mg	☐ 5 mg	40 mg	50 mg
Ritalin (methylphe-nidate HCl)	10, 20 mg tab	5 mg b.i.d. to t.i.d., con-sider q.i.d.	☐ 5–10 mg	☐ 5–10 mg	60 mg	100 mg

Table 11.1 Medical treatment, continued

BRAND NAME (ACTIVE CHEMICAL)	DOSAGE FORM	START-ING DOSE	TITRATION SCHEDULE EVERY 7 DAYS		MAXIMUM DAILY* (>70 KG)[1,2]	
			As per product mono-graph	As per CAD-DRA board	As per product mono-graph	As per CAD-DRA board
Ritalin SR[7] (methylphe-nidate HCl)	20 mg tab	20 mg q.d. a.m.	☐ 20 mg (add q2pm dose)	☐ 20 mg (add q2pm dose)	60 mg	100 mg

** Indications for use: a) p.r.n. for particular activities; b) to augment long-acting for-mulations early or late in the day, or early in the evening and c) when LA agents are cost prohibitive. To augment Adderall XR® or Vyvanse®, short-acting and intermediate-acting dextro-amphetamine products can be used. To augment Biphentin® or Concerta® short-acting MPH products can be used. b.i.d. refers to qam and qnoon and t.i.d. refers to qam, qnoon and q4pm points.

[6] Dexedrine Spansule may last 6–8 hours.

[7] Ritalin SR may help cover the noon period but clinical experience suggests an effect simi-lar to short-acting preparations.

Generic medications

PMS or Ratio-meth-ylphenidate	5, 10, 20 mg tab	10 mg q.d. a.m. and noon	☐ 10 mg	☐ 10 mg	72 mg	100 mg
			(add q4pm dose)			
Novo-MPH ER-C	18, 27, 36, 54 mg tab	18 mg q.d. a.m. and noon	☐ 18 mg/ wk	☐ 18 mg/ wk	54 mg	108 mg

Reproduced with permission from the Canadian Attention Deficit Hyperactivity Disorder Resource Alliance *Canadian ADHD Practice Guidelines*, 2nd Edition (Turgay et al., 2011).

· **Group interventions**: If possible, establish a group of adult patients because it is helpful to them to learn from each other and it is cost-effective in seeing many patients with similar problems at the same time. This may be difficult to implement if space is an issue, so it may be necessary to outsource this activity.

· **Individual therapy**: Cognitive-behavioural therapy, as would be expected given the relationship of ADHD to mood disorders, is very useful in helping to reframe many of the negative situations into positive ones. ADHD patients have belief systems based on a lack of accomplishment and, at times, a cynical worldview where everyone else is doing well and they are not, given their potential. They need the encouragement of their clinician that ultimately helps to create greater self-control. It is here that primary care clinicians have their greatest influence, as the therapeutic long-term alliance is the anchor of stability that the patient seeks.

When to refer to a specialist

Unfortunately, finding someone who specializes in adult ADHD is often difficult or impossible, depending on where your practice is. Few psychiatrists understand or specialize in this condition, which means that treatment is most often carried out in primary care. However, this is slowly changing.

Consider making a referral when the patient has:

· comorbid conditions that require multiple medications to treat
· complicated medical problems that may require a multi-specialty approach, though the primary care may be useful in co-ordinating treatment
· side-effects to their current medical treatment that require management (e.g., sleep problems, problems with memory, etc.)
· various medico-legal or advocacy situations that are beyond the expertise of primary care clinicians (e.g., application for disability claims, job-related conflicts, assessments of learning, etc.)
· failure to respond as desired to a medication after a trial period.

Outcome

People with ADHD can function well if they can find appropriate interventions to contain their disorder. The ideal situation is if the attributes of their disorder are used in a productive capacity. Impulsivity becomes entrepreneurship and opportunism, inattention becomes inventiveness and broad thinking, and motor hyperactivity becomes physical stamina and drive. Many ADHD patients have highly successful careers as a result. This should be the motivation of the clinician to identify the disorder properly and to seek effective treatment.

Community and online resources

Canadian ADHD Resource Alliance: CADDRA is an affiliation of physicians who assess and treat patients with ADHD in Canada. CADDRA provides:
- a free hard copy of the *Canadian ADHD Practice Guidelines* to CADDRA members (non-members can order a copy): www.caddra.ca
- online username-password access to questionnaire scoring programs
- access to mentorship and consultants across the country.
- Centre for ADD/ADHD Advocacy, Canada (www.caddac.ca). Provides help for parents of children with ADHD.
· Teach ADHD (www.teachADHD.ca). Provides information for educators.
· Totally ADD (www.totallyadd.com) is a Canadian web site for adults with ADD, created by actor and comedian Rick Green and full of engaging, humorous videos.
· American Academy of Child and Adolescent Psychiatry (www.aacap.org). Provides links to the practice parameters for ADHD.

References

American Psychiatric Association. (2000). *Diagnostic and Statistical Manual of Mental Disorders* (4th ed., text rev.). Washington DC: Author.

Biederman, J., Faraone, S.V., Spencer, T., Wilens, T., Norman, D., Lapey, K.A. et al. (1993). Patterns of psychiatric comorbidity, cognition and psychosocial functioning in adults with attention deficit hyperactivity disorder. *American Journal of Psychiatry, 50* (12), 1792–1798.

Kessler, R.C., Adler, L., Ames, M., Demler, O., Faraone, S., Hiripi, E. et al. (2005). The World Health Organization adult ADHD self-report scale (ASRS): A short screening scale for use in the general population. *Psychological Medicine, 35* (2), 245–256. DOI: 10.1017/S0033291704002892

Murphy, K. & Barkley, R.A. (1996). Parents of children with ADHD: Psychological and attentional impairment. *American Journal of Orthopsychiatry, 66* (1), 93–102.

Turgay, A., Jain, U. & Bedard, A. (2011). *Canadian ADHD Practice Guidelines* (2nd ed.). Toronto: McCleery-McCann Health Care.

Weiss, G. & Hechtman, L.T. (1993). *Hyperactive Children Grown Up: ADHD in Children, Adolescents, and Adults* (2nd ed.). New York: Guildford Press.

12

The patient with a sleep disorder

COLIN SHAPIRO, M.R. GOOLAM HUSSAIN AND DORA ZALAI

Introduction

Sleep disorders are common and have profound neurocognitive, cardiovascular, therapeutic and safety ramifications. Research has demonstrated that sleep is a restorative process and that lack of sleep or disruption of sleep will have many implications, including:

- high rates of fatigue (a more common presenting symptom of sleep disorder than sleepiness *per se*)
- cardiac and vascular complications
- higher risk of driving accidents
- compromised immune function
- more rapid deterioration in many medical conditions due to disrupted sleep.

This last observation regarding the deterioration of medical conditions is of particular relevance to the primary care provider because managing sleep problems represents a valuable opportunity for intervention. Furthermore, there is evidence that sleep disorders may prevent the full action of medical treatments for hypertension, cardiac failure, mood disorders and epilepsy. In children with an underlying and easily treatable sleep disorder, the erroneous diagnosis of attention-deficit/hyperactivity disorder will hinder recovery and have an impact on academic performance, socialization and long-term function. For all these reasons, a clear perspective of the requirements of assessing and managing sleep problems is vital, particularly as most clinicians have received little to no training in sleep medicine, which has advanced enormously over the last 20 to 30 years.

Description of the problem

Although there are currently more than 80 different sleep disorders recognized, the old European simplistic classification of problems of too little sleep (insomnia), problems of too much sleep (hypersomnia, excessive sleepiness), circadian rhythm problems and "things that go bump in the night" (parasomnias), is a useful rubric for classifying symptoms and management. We will focus on insomnia and excessive sleepiness in this chapter since these are the most common presenting complaints in primary care.

Insomnia is defined as a persistent difficulty falling asleep or staying asleep, awakening earlier than the person wishes or having non-restorative sleep despite adequate circumstances for sleep. Acute insomnia lasts for less than a month and is usually triggered by acute medical illness or stress. Chronic insomnia persists for more than 30 days and, if untreated, often lasts for decades.

Excessive sleepiness is characterized by a complaint of constant or recurrent daytime sleepiness, typically with inappropriate sleep episodes.

Making the diagnosis: The key clinical questions and screening tools

Insomnia

The Athens Insomnia Scale (Soldatos et al., 2000) is a self-report questionnaire that patients can complete in five minutes in the clinician's office (see page 210). If the person scores a total higher than 10 (Soldatos et al., 2003), assess the following:

SLEEP SCHEDULE AND SLEEP HYGIENE
Collect information on bedtime, the time it takes them to fall asleep, the number and duration of nighttime awakenings, the final awakening in the morning, the time they get out of bed and the difference between weeknight and weekend sleep schedule and sleep quality. Learn about bedtime routine and any disturbing factors in the sleep environment such as television, computers or telephones.

ANXIETY OR WORRY AT NIGHT
Ask patients about anxiety, worry, frustration, problem-solving, rumination about stressful issues, inability to "switch off" their mind when they are lying awake in bed at night.

DAYTIME FUNCTIONING
Assess daytime sleepiness, mental and physical fatigue, problems with concentration and memory and inquire about mood and irritability. Daytime sleepiness is usually not the leading daytime symptom of insomnia; patients more often complain about mental exhaustion and an inability to nap during the day.

MEDICAL DISORDERS
Screen for specific sleep disorders, medical and psychiatric conditions that may cause insomnia (see "Differential diagnosis: Insomnia," page 213).

MEDICATIONS
Review medications that have a CNS-stimulating effect or disrupt sleep (e.g., diuretics).

SUBSTANCE USE
Inquire about caffeine and other substance use; consider alcohol withdrawal.

Excessive sleepiness: Screening for apnea
The most common daytime symptoms of sleep disorders are daytime sleepiness and fatigue. All patients who are tired, sleepy or fatigued should be screened for sleep apnea.

The Athens Insomnia Scale

This scale is intended to record your own assessment of any sleep difficulty you might have experienced. Please check (by circling the appropriate number) the items below to indicate your estimate of any difficulty, provided that it occurred at least three times per week during the last month.

SLEEP INDUCTION (TIME IT TAKES YOU TO FALL ASLEEP AFTER TURNING OFF THE LIGHTS)

| 0: No problem | 1: Slightly delayed | 2: Markedly delayed | 3: Very delayed or did not sleep at all |

AWAKENINGS DURING THE NIGHT

| 0: No problem | 1: Minor problem | 2: Considerable problem | 3: Serious problem or did not sleep at all |

FINAL AWAKENING EARLIER THAN DESIRED

| 0: Not earlier | 1: A little earlier | 2: Markedly earlier | 3: Much earlier or did not sleep at all |

TOTAL SLEEP DURATION

| 0: Sufficient | 1: Slightly insufficient | 2: Markedly insufficient | 3: Very insufficient or did not sleep at all |

OVERALL QUALITY OF SLEEP (NO MATTER HOW LONG YOU SLEPT)

| 0: Satisfactory | 1: Slightly unsatisfactory | 2: Markedly unsatisfactory | 3: Very unsatisfactory or did not sleep at all |

SENSE OF WELL-BEING DURING THE DAY

| 0: Normal | 1: Slightly decreased | 2: Markedly decreased | 3: Very decreased |

FUNCTIONING (PHYSICAL AND MENTAL) DURING THE DAY

0: Normal	1: Slightly de-creased	2: Markedly decreased	3: Very decreased

SLEEPINESS DURING THE DAY

0: None	1: Mild	2: Considerable	3: Intense

Maximum score: 24; Threshold for insomnia: 10 (Soldatos et al., 2003).

Reproduced with permission, copyright Constantin Soldatos, 2000.

A short questionnaire to assess excessive sleepiness is the Epworth Sleepiness Scale (see page 212). Most patients can complete the scale in two to three minutes. A score of nine or more is considered a positive score for sleepiness.

A simple screening tool to detect sleep apnea is STOP, a mnemonic that stands for the following questions:
· Do you **S**nore?
· Do you feel **T**ired, fatigued or sleepy during the day?
· Has anyone **O**bserved you stop breathing in your sleep?
· Do you have high blood **P**ressure?

If the answers to two of the four STOP questions are positive there is a 77 per cent chance of the person having apnea. If the person has a positive STOP screen, the additional mnemonic BANG may also need to be considered.
· BMI: >35
· Age: >50 years
· Neck circumference: >40 cm
· Gender: male

The sensitivity of the STOP and BANG screening questions for mild, moderate and severe sleep apnea are 84 per cent, 97 per cent and 100 per cent respectively.

Epworth Sleepiness Scale

How likely are you to doze off or fall asleep in the following situations, in contrast to feeling just tired? This refers to your usual way of life in recent times. Even if you have not done some of these things recently, try to work out how they would have affected you. Use the following scale to choose the most appropriate number for each situation:

0 = would never doze   2 = moderate chance of dozing
1 = slight chance of dozing   3 = high chance of dozing

SITUATION	CHANCE OF DOZING			
	0	1	2	3
1. Sitting and reading	0	1	2	3
2. Watching TV	0	1	2	3
3. Sitting, inactive in a public place (e.g., theatre or a meeting)	0	1	2	3
4. As a passenger in a car for an hour without a break	0	1	2	3
5. Lying down to rest in the afternoon when circumstances permit	0	1	2	3
6. Sitting and talking to someone	0	1	2	3
7. Sitting quietly after a lunch without alcohol	0	1	2	3
8. In a car, while stopped for a few minutes in the traffic	0	1	2	3

Scoring:
1–6: Congratulations, you are getting enough sleep!
7–8: Your score is average.
9 and up: Very sleepy and should seek medical advice.

Reproduced with permission. Copyright, M.W. Johns, 1990, 1997.

Differential diagnosis

Insomnia

The presumptive cause of insomnia can be thought of as the five Ps:

1. **P**hysical causes may relate to the bedroom environment; for example, noise, light, temperature or television.

2. **P**sychophysiological refers to the development of insomnia after a stressful life event. For example, following bereavement all the features of the bereavement resolve but the sleep disturbance may persist.

3. **P**sychological/psychiatric cause of initial insomnia is typically anxiety. Maintenance insomnia (disrupted sleep) occurs in many psychiatric disorders, including eating disorders, dementia and schizophrenia. Terminal insomnia (early morning awakenings) is most characteristic of depression.

4. **P**athophysiological insomnia describes medical conditions comorbid with insomnia. These conditions range from pain conditions, including fibromyalgia and arthritis, to hyperthyroidism, to respiratory and cardiac disorders including emphysema and congestive heart failure. They also include conditions affecting the central nervous system such as dementia, head injuries, Parkinson's disease and organ failure and specific sleep disorders such as obstructive sleep apnea and periodic leg movement in sleep.

5. **P**harmacological causes, which are related to the use of medications such as antidepressants, stimulants, antihypertensives including beta blockers, decongestants and corticosteroids. Also consider the rebound effect of the withdrawal of sedating agents including alcohol and short-acting hypnotics.

Excessive daytime sleepiness

Causes of excessive daytime sleepiness that should be considered include the following:

SLEEP RESTRICTION

Sleep restriction (insufficient sleep) is the most common cause of excessive daytime sleepiness in healthy individuals.

SLEEP APNEA

People with sleep apnea (see pages 209–211 for screening information) stop breathing at least five times per hour for greater than 10-second periods due to upper airway occlusion (obstructive sleep apnea) or the cessation of the respiratory effort (central sleep apnea). Although patients with sleep apnea may apparently sleep through the night, their sleep is fragmented by short arousals following apneic episodes and becomes devoid of a sense of having refreshing sleep. People with sleep apnea often complain of morning headaches and daytime fatigue and feel tired when they wake up from naps.

NARCOLEPSY

The leading symptom of narcolepsy, a rare condition that is genetic or posttraumatic in origin, is excessive daytime sleepiness with short (10–20 minute) naps, or sudden, irresistible sleep attacks from which patients wake up refreshed. Patients may also experience cataplexy (loss of muscle tone in strong emotional states), sleep paralysis (brief inability to move from awakenings) and sleep-related hallucinations.

PERIODIC LIMB MOVEMENT DISORDER

Periodic limb movement disorder (PLMS), repeated twitches of the legs in sleep, is more common in the elderly population, in vertebral degenerative disorders, in women who are pregnant, in patients with Parkinson's disease and in those with chronic kidney disease. It also occurs with low ferritin and with vitamin B12 deficiency states. PLMS may be problematic even at the lower end of normal range for ferritin levels.

SUBSTANCE USE OR USE OF MEDICATIONS

The use of drugs such as benzodiazepines and antihistamines, alcohol and withdrawal from stimulants should be considered.

MEDICAL DISORDERS

Acute, systemic infections are a common cause of excessive daytime sleepiness. Neurological disorders (infections, epilepsy, posttrauma) and metabolic disorders affecting the central nervous system are also often associated with excessive daytime sleepiness.

PSYCHIATRIC DISORDERS
Although depression is usually comorbid with insomnia, 20 per cent of patients who are depressed describe fatigue and excessive sleepiness. Atypical depression is characterized by hypersomnia. Posttraumatic stress disorder may induce pathological sleep architecture and cause fragmented sleep depriving patients of restorative sleep.

CIRCADIAN RHYTHM DISORDERS
Circadian rhythm disorders are defined as a discrepancy between the person's sleep schedule and the schedule that is considered the norm for school, work or other obligations. The most common circadian problem in primary care involves patients who are shift workers.

A common problem in adolescents is the delayed sleep phase syndrome (DSPS). In DSPS, the sleep-wake cycle is shifted to early morning bedtime and mid-day wake-up time. Teenagers with DSPS have difficulty getting up in the morning on school days and suffer from sleepiness until the afternoon.

MISCELLANEOUS CONDITIONS
Other conditions than can be considered include idiopathic hypersomnia, post-viral hypersomnia, genetic causes and Kleine-Levin syndrome (adolescent hyperphagia, aggression and hypersexuality).

Treatment options

Insomnia

PSYCHOEDUCATION
Education about normal sleep and sleep hygiene issues is an essential part of insomnia and sleep treatment. Information that should be discussed with patients includes:
· the average and individual sleep need
· the change of sleep need with age
· the circadian rhythm
· the importance of a regular sleep schedule

- the role of napping in compensating for lost sleep contributing to the perpetuation of chronic insomnia
- the consequences of sleep deprivation
- the effect of caffeine, nicotine, medications and alcohol on sleep.

There are specific behavioural techniques to help consolidate sleep (bed restriction) and strategies for helping withdraw patients from long-term hypnotic drug use. The use of actigraphy (a portable device used to assess sleep/wake patterns and circadian rhythms) can be useful for these behavioural therapies.

COGNITIVE-BEHAVIOURAL THERAPY (CBT)

Cognitive-behavioural therapy (CBT) addresses the maladaptive behaviours and dysfunctional beliefs that sustain insomnia. According to the cognitive-behavioural model of insomnia, people with acute insomnia adopt behavioural strategies, and cultivate sleep-related anxiety, which are fuelled by unhelpful cognitions about sleep. These, independent of the cause of the insomnia, perpetuate the condition. CBT is a short treatment (commonly five to eight sessions) that is beneficial for many patients suffering from insomnia, and which can be administered alone or in combination with hypnotics. Since it eliminates maladaptive behaviours and cognitions, it provides improvements that endure well beyond the termination of active treatment.

PHARMACOTHERAPY

Sleep-promoting agents (hypnotics or sedatives) are generally recommended for short-term treatment of insomnia. Some sedating agents have the potential for physical or psychological dependence and there are limited studies on the effects of long-term hypnotic use. For the available range of pharmacotherapies for sleep disorders, see Table 12.1 on page 218.

In situations where insomnia presents with another illness, insomnia should be considered a comorbid condition rather than simply a manifestation of the other illness. As such, the insomnia should be specifically targeted for treatment. It is important to emphasize that taking a hypnotic does not decrease the need for psychoeducation and cognitive-behavioural intervention.

Similarly, long-term hypnotic use should not be denied to a patient if the patient is clearly benefitting. The cost—benefit balance needs to include an awareness of, for example, the fact that patients with insomnia have twice the rate of motor vehicle accidents; however, as with all long-term treatments, monitoring and re-evaluating the underlying condition should be stringent and may be best done in a specialized clinic.

Most current hypnotics/sedatives are more effective for the symptomatic treatment of sleep-initiation insomnia than for sleep-maintenance insomnia. Some novel medications have been developed specifically for the treatment of insomnia while others have been used in the past decades because of their sedative side-effects. The former include the "Z-drugs"—zopiclone, zaleplon and zolpidem—and the melatonin receptor agonist ramelteon. Of these, only zopiclone (Imovane) is currently available in Canada although zaleplon can be obtained from a compounding pharmacy. With the appearance of these specific hypnotics, the benzodiazepines have become less commonly prescribed for insomnia. Recently L-tryptophan (Tryptan), an essential amino acid and the precursor of serotonin, has been increasingly used. The use of hypnotics in children is viewed as less desirable and a parsimonious solution is to use tryptophan at an increasing dosage to gain a hypnotic effect. Melatonin is a hormone produced in the pineal gland with a strong chronobiotic and a less pronounced hypnotic effect. It is the first choice treatment of delayed sleep phase syndrome especially if the impaired melatonin production is proven by a specific (dim light melatonin onset) test. Although used widely as a hypnotic, this unregulated use does not take into account potential risk of melatonin use especially in younger patients. There is no other hormone so casually prescribed as melatonin.

TREATMENT OF EXCESSIVE DAYTIME SLEEPINESS
The pharmacological (and other) treatment of excessive sleepiness should be specific to the underlying problem. The paradoxical use of a hypnotic, if there is no other specific cause for excessive sleepiness other than repeated, spontaneous arousals recorded at the sleep lab, can be useful. The best approach is often a course of treatment lasting two months with a review approximately two to four weeks after cessation of the medication.

Table 12.1 Pharmacotherapies for sleep disorders

CLASS NAME (TRADE NAME)	HALF LIFE, DOSE AND RANGE	POSITIVES	NEGATIVES
Benzodiazepine			
Temazepam (Restoril)	5–20 hours 15 and 30 mg Maximum/ 24 hours: 60 mg	• Initial insomnia • Less hang-over effect	• Withdrawals • Addiction and dependence • Tolerance • Pregnancy and breastfeeding • Elderly
Lorazepam (Ativan)	10–20 hours 0.5, 1.0 and 2.0 mg Maximum/ 24 hours: 4 mg	• Insomnia • Anxiety • Safe in liver disease	• Withdrawal • Addiction and dependence • Tolerance • Pregnancy and breast-feeding • Elderly
Oxazepam (Serax)	5–15 hours 10, 15 and 30 mg Maximum/ 24 hours: 30 mg)	• Anxiety • Alcohol withdrawal • Safe in liver disease	• Withdrawal • Addiction and dependence • Tolerance • Pregnancy and breast-feeding • Elderly

DRUG INTERACTION	BEST USED FOR	SIDE-EFFECTS
• CNS depressants	• Insomnia • Muscle relaxant	• Behaviour changes • Confusion • Irritability • Balance issues • Drowsiness • Increased nervousness • Mood changes • Worsening of sleep apnea • Withdrawal • Seizure • Headache • REM suppression
• CNS depressants • Divalproex • Phenytoin • Theophylline • Co-administration of IM benzodiazepine and IM olanzapine	• Anxiety disorder • Seizure disorder • Insomnia	• Anterograde amnesia • Confusion • Behavioural changes • Irritability • Increased nervousness • Mood changes • Withdrawal, seizure • Headaches • Balance and fall issues
• CNS depressants • Co-adminstration of IM benzodiazepine and IM olanzapine • Phenytoin • Theophylline	• Anxiety • Alcohol withdrawal	• Anterograde amnesia • Confusion • Behavioural changes • Irritability • Increased nervousness • Mood changes • Withdrawal, seizure • Headaches • Balance and fall issues

Table 12.1 Pharmacotherapies, continued

CLASS NAME (TRADE NAME)	HALF LIFE, DOSE AND RANGE	POSITIVES	NEGATIVES
Alprazolam (Xanax)	6–12 hours 0.25 mg, 0.5 mg, 2 mg Maximum/ 24 hours: 6 mg	• Helpful for anxiety attacks	• Withdrawals • Addiction and dependence • Tolerance • Pregnancy and breastfeeding • Elderly
Clonazepam (Rivotril)	18–50 hours 0.5 mg and 2 mg Maximum/ 24 hours: 4 mg	• Insomnia • Anxiety • Restless legs syndrome	• Withdrawals • Addiction and dependence • Tolerance • Pregnancy and breastfeeding. • Narrow angle glaucoma • Liver disease • Kidney disease • Sensitivity to diazepam • Elderly
Diazepam (Valium)	20–100 hours 5 mg, 10 mg Maximum/ 24 hours: 40 mg	• Status epilepticus • Alcohol withdrawal • Sedation for certain procedures such as endoscopies • Fewer withdrawal effects	• Addiction and dependence • Tolerance • Pregnancy and breastfeeding • Narrow angle glaucoma • Liver disease • Kidney disease • Elderly • Respiratory disease • Overdose • Coma

DRUG INTERACTION	BEST USED FOR	SIDE-EFFECTS
• CNS depressants • Imipramine and Desipramine • CYP3A inhibitors and inducers	• Generalized anxiety disorder • Panic attacks • Muscle relaxant • Depression • PTSD	• Short acting • Behaviour changes • Confusion • Irritability • Balance issues, falls • Drowsiness • Increased nervousness • Mood changes • Worsening of sleep apnea • Withdrawals, seizure • Headache
• CNS depressants • Opioids • Antihistamine • Disulfiram • Phenobarbital • Phenytoin • Carbamazepine • Theophylline • Rifampicin	• Insomnia • Periodic limb movements • Status epileptics • Anxiety disorder	• Fatigue • Sexual dysfunction • Behaviour changes • Confusion, irritability • Balance issues • Drowsiness • Increased nervousness • Mood changes • Worsening of sleep apnea • Withdrawals, seizure • Headache • REM suppression
• Barbiturates • Phenothiazines • Narcotics • Antidepressants • Agents that have an effect on hepatic cytochrome P450	• Status epilepticus • Alcohol withdrawal • Eclampsia • Anxiety • Panic attack • Agitation • Muscle relaxant • Sedation for preoperative reasons • Insomnia	• Slow elimination • Behaviour changes, confusion • Irritability • Balance issues • Drowsiness • Increased nervousness • Mood changes • Worsening of sleep apnea • Withdrawals, seizure • Headache • REM suppression

Table 12.1 Pharmacotherapies, continued

CLASS NAME (TRADE NAME)	HALF LIFE, DOSE AND RANGE	POSITIVES	NEGATIVES
Bromazepam (Lectopam)	10–20 hours 1 mg, 3 mg, 6 mg Maximum/ 24 hours: 6–9 mg	• Initial insomnia	• Withdrawals • Addiction and dependence • Tolerance • Pregnancy and breastfeeding • Narrow angle glaucoma • Liver disease • Kidney disease • Sensitivity to diazepam • Elderly • Overdose
Cannabanoid			
Nabilone (Cesamet)	2–35 hours 0.5 mg Maximum/ 24 hours: 1 mg	• Antiemetic • Neuro- pathic pain	• Liver disease • Hypertension • Heart disease • Mania • Schizophrenia • Allergy to compound • Addiction • Pregnancy • Elderly • Breastfeeding • Overdose

DRUG INTERACTION	BEST USED FOR	SIDE-EFFECTS
• Fluvoxamine • Cimetidine • Propranolol	• Anxiolytic • Hypnotic at a high dose	• Behaviour changes • Confusion, irritability • Balance issues • Drowsiness • Increased nervousness • Mood changes • Withdrawals, seizure • Headache
• Anticholinergic • Naltrexone • Theophylline • Antihistamine • Barbiturate • Benzodiazapine • Carbamazepine • Codeine • Zolpidem • Chlorpromazine • Risperidone • Trazodone • Cough medications	• Neuropathic pain • Fibromyalgia • Movement disorders • Antiemetic for cancer chemotherapy • Chronic pain	• Dizziness • Dryness of mouth • Euphoria • Headache • Sleep disturbance • Memory problems • Mood changes • Confusion

Table 12.1 Pharmacotherapies, continued

CLASS NAME (TRADE NAME)	HALF LIFE, DOSE AND RANGE	POSITIVES	NEGATIVES
Sedating antidepressant			
Mirtazapine (Remeron)	20–40 hours 15 mg, 30 mg Maximum/ 24 hours: up to 60–120 mg	• Sedating; promotes slow wave sleep • Antidepressant • Anxiolytic	• Weight gain
Clomipramine (Anafranil)	21 hours 25 mg or 75 mg SR Maximum/ 24 hours: 300 mg	• No addiction • Sedation	• Withdrawals • Pregnancy • Breastfeeding • Overdose • Closed angle glaucoma • Seizures • Cardiovascular (premature ventricular contractions, ST changes) • Blood pressure change
Trazodone (Desryel)	5–9 hours 25 mg, 50 mg Maximum/ 24 hours: 600 mg	• Anxiolytic and hypnotic, less prominent anticholinergic and sexual side-effects	• Pregnancy • Lactation • Overdose

DRUG INTERACTION	BEST USED FOR	SIDE-EFFECTS
• Alcohol • Barbiturates • Carbamazepine • Cimetidine • Erythromycin • Warfarin	• Depression • Insomnia • Anxiety disorders	• Dizziness • Dryness of mouth • Euphoria • Headache • Somnolence • Weight gain • Increased libido • Constipation • Vivid dreams
• MAO inhibitors • CNS stimulants • SSRI • Tranquilizers • Narcotics • Alcohol • Antihypertensive • Cold medications • St. John's wort	• Obsessive-compulsive disorder • Depression • Panic disorder • Narcolepsy (cataplexy) • Insomnia • Premature ejaculation • Depersonalization • Panic disorder • Enuresis • Chronic pain • Reduce relapse in cocaine addiction	• Dizziness • Dryness of mouth • Euphoria • Headache • Somnolence • Weight gain • Increased libido • Constipation • Vivid dreams • Agitation, increased anxiety • Anticholinergic • Antiadrenergic side-effects • Sexual problems • Hypersensitivity reaction
• CYP3A4 inhibitors • CNS depressant	• Depression, bipolar disorder • Fibromyalgia • Sleep disturbance • Panic disorder • Diabetic neuropathy • Complex pain syndrome • Alcohol withdrawal • Eating disorder	• Fatigue • Lethargy, psychomotor retardation • Confusion • Memory loss • Priapism • Tremors • Headache • Hypertension • Tachycardia, bradycardia, palpitation • Nausea, vomiting • Hypersensitivity reaction

Table 12.1 Pharmacotherapies, continued

CLASS NAME (TRADE NAME)	HALF LIFE, DOSE AND RANGE	POSITIVES	NEGATIVES
Melatonin receptor agonist			
Ramelteon	0.8–2.6 hours Maximum/ 24 hours: 8 mg	• Initial insomnia	• Hypersensitivity to remelteon or any of its product ingredients • Caution with hepatic impairment
Tryptophan			
Tryptophan (Tryptan)	— 750 mg Maximum/ 24 hours: 4500 mg	• Promotes slow wave sleep • Natural food substance • Insomnia	• Hypersensitivity • Do not use after protein-rich meal
Z drugs			
Zolpidem (Ambien, Ambien CR, Stilnox)	2–6 hours 5 and 10 mg, 6.25 and 12.5 mg extended release —	• Initial insomnia • Less rebound insomnia • Less risk of dependence	• Not available in Canada
Zopiclone (Imovane)	3.5–6.5 hours 7.5 mg, 5 mg Maximum/ 24 hours: 15 mg	• Does not disrupt sleep architecture • Initial and middle insomnia • Less addictive	• Taste side-effect • Addiction and withdrawal • Rebound insomnia • Abuse • Seizures

DRUG INTERACTION	BEST USED FOR	SIDE-EFFECTS
• Fluvoxamine	• Sleep onset insomnia	• Headache • Somnolence • Fatigue • Nausea • Dizziness • Insomnia
• Vitamin B6 • Citalopram	• Insomnia • Pain syndrome	• Nausea • Vomiting • Headache • Palpitation • Agitation
• Chropromazine • Fluconazole • Imipramine • Rifampacin • Carbamazepine • Phenytoin	• Initial insomnia	• Nausea, vomiting • Headache • Palpitation • Agitation • Anterograde amnesia, delusions • Impaired judgment and reasoning
• Carbamazepine • Phenytoin • Erythromycin • Rifampicin • Ketoconozole • Imipramine	• Initial, middle and late insomnia	• Gustatory side-effect • Somnolence • Confusion, memory impairment • Headache, dizziness, fatigue • Mood changes • Nausea

Table 12.1 Pharmacotherapies, continued

CLASS NAME (TRADE NAME)	HALF LIFE, DOSE AND RANGE	POSITIVES	NEGATIVES
Zaleplon (Starnoc)	1–4 hours 10 mg —	• Maintenance insomnia • Less risk of dependence • Rebound insomnia • No hangover	• Short acting • Abuse • Not routinely available in Canada
Melatonin			
Melatonin	Unknown 2 mg, 3 mg Maximum/ 24 hours: 3–6 mg	• Phase delay syndrome • Circadian rhythm disorder • Shift work	• None
Antihistamine			
Diphenhydramine (Benadryl)	Short 25 mg, 50 mg Maximum/ 24 hours: 50 mg	• Sedative • Anti-allergy	• Addiction • To be used with caution in children and in patients with lung disease • Blood pressure • Narrow angle glaucoma • Heart disease • Asthma

DRUG INTERACTION	BEST USED FOR	SIDE-EFFECTS
• Cimetidine • Rifampicin • Thioridazine	• Middle of night insomnia	• Confusion • Drowsiness, dizziness • Headache • Nausea, vomiting • Tremors • Memory problem
• Unknown	• Circadian rhythm disorder	• Drowsiness • Fatigue
• Alcohol • Anticholinergic • Narcotics • Tranquilizers • Antipsychotic	• Anti-allergy • Cough medication	• Drowsiness • Confusion • Dry mouth • Appetite changes • Headache • Restlessness

Table 12.1 Pharmacotherapies, continued

CLASS NAME (TRADE NAME)	HALF LIFE, DOSE AND RANGE	POSITIVES	NEGATIVES
Chloral hydrate			
Chloral hydrate	4–12 hours Adults: 500 to 1 000 mg, 15 to 30 minutes before bedtime. Geriatrics: Initial 250 mg, 15 to 30 minutes before bedtime. Children: 50 mg/kg at bedtime, maximum 1 000 mg per single dose	• Short-term treatment of insomnia • Sedative prior to EEG does not suppress epileptiform discharges • No REM rebound • Alcohol withdrawal	• Suppresses respiration and blood pressure • Kidney disease • Liver disease • Heart and stomach problems • Pregnancy, breastfeeding • Asthma • Overdose • Abuse • Withdrawal
Antipsychotic			
Quetiapine (Seroquel)	6 hours 25 mg, 50 mg, 100 mg Maximum/ 24 hours: 25–100 mg for insomnia	• Peak plasma level 1.5 hours, fast acting	• Morning sedation • Acts at multiple receptors (adrenergic, muscarinic, serotonergic, dopaminergic) • Not many studies done for insomnia

DRUG INTERACTION	BEST USED FOR	SIDE-EFFECTS
• Anticoagulant • Antihistamine • Furosemide (Lasix) • Seizure medication • Antidepressant • Sleeping pills	• Short-term insomnia • Prior to dental surgery • Alcohol withdrawal	• Drowsiness • Upset stomach, vomiting, diarrhea
• Drug interaction related to enzyme induction and inhibition	• Antipsychotic • Mood stabilizer	• Agitation • Weight gain • Metabolic side-effects • Tardive dyskinesia • Drowsiness, confusion • Dry mouth • Appetite changes • Headache • Restlessness

Table 12.1 Pharmacotherapies, continued

CLASS NAME (TRADE NAME)	HALF LIFE, DOSE AND RANGE	POSITIVES	NEGATIVES
Olanzapine (Zyprexa)	20–50 hours 2.5 mg, 5 mg, 10 mg Maximu/ 24 hours: 15 mg for insomnia	• Sedating	• Hangover in the morning • Metabolic side-effects • Acts at multiple receptors (adren-ergic, muscarinic, serotonergic, dopaminergic) • Not many studies done for insomnia

When to refer to a sleep specialist

Insomnia

Most cases of insomnia can be reliably assessed and effectively treated in primary care. In cases in which a five-to-eight session course of CBT or a seven-day pharmacological treatment does not relieve the symptoms, referral to a sleep specialist is recommended.

Sleepiness

If the problem of sleepiness and fatigue is clearly related to sleep restriction, suggest that the patient enter into a contract of giving increased time for sleep on a regular basis. Suggest a trial period of one month with a clear benefit in terms of resolving the underlying problem.

DRUG INTERACTION	BEST USED FOR	SIDE-EFFECTS
• Drug interaction related to enzyme induction and inhibition	• Antipsychotic • Mood stabilizer • Sedation	• Weight gain • Metabolic side-effects more than Seroquel • Drowsiness • Confusion • Dry mouth • Appetite changes • Headache • Restlessness

Patients with excessive sleepiness should be referred for a more formal sleep assessment at a sleep clinic.

Recommended books and websites for patients and health professionals

The website of the Sleep and Alertness Clinic at Toronto Western Hospital (www.sleepontario.com) provides detailed information on sleep disorders for patients and health care professionals, free downloadable leaflets for health care professionals on a wide range of sleep disorders and treatment options, information on ongoing research projects and a comprehensive collection of articles and books on sleep. The website www.sleeplab.ca also provides valuable detailed information for primary care providers.

People with insomnia can use *Overcoming Insomnia: A Cognitive-Behavioral Therapy Approach* (Oxford, 2008) as a self-help treatment guide or as a workbook in therapist-guided treatment. A manual for clinicians is also available with the same title.

References

Buysse, D.J., Germain, A., Moul, D.E., Franzen, P.L., Brar, L.K. et al. (2011). Efficacy of brief behavioral treatment for chronic insomnia in older adults. *Archives of Internal Medicine, 171*, 887–895.

Chung, F., Yegneswaran, B., Liao, P., Chung, S.A., Vairavanathan, S., Islam, S. et al. (2008). STOP questionnaire: A tool to screen patients for obstructive sleep apnea. *Anesthesiology, 108* (5), 812–821. DOI: 10.1097/ALN.0b013e31816d83e4

Edinger, J.D. & Carney, C.E. (2008). *Overcoming Insomnia: A Cognitive-Behavioral Therapy Approach Workbook*. New York: Oxford University Press.

Johns, M. (1991). A new method for measuring daytime sleepiness: The Epworth Sleepiness Scale. *Sleep, 14* (6), 540–545.

Soldatos, C.R., Dikeos, D.G. & Paparrigopoulos, T.J. (2000). Athens Insomnia Scale: Validation of an instrument based on ICD-10 criteria. *Journal of Psychosomatic Research. 48* (6), 550–560. DOI: 10.1016/S0022-3999(00)00095-7

Soldatos, C.R., Dikeos, D.G. & Paparrigopoulos, T.J. (2003). The diagnostic validity of the Athens Insomnia Scale. *Journal of Psychosomatic Research. 55* (3), 263–267. DOI: 10.1016/S0022-3999(02)00604-9

Special topics

13

Assessment and management of suicide risk

MARILYN A. CRAVEN, PAUL S. LINKS AND GREGOR NOVAK

Epidemiology of suicide in Canada

- More than 3,600 people die by suicide in Canada each year (10.8/100,000).
- Men die by suicide three to four times more often than women; however, women are three to four times more likely to attempt suicide.
- Suicide rates are higher in young people aged 15 to 24 and in elderly males, compared to the general population (Canadian Association for Suicide Prevention, 2009).

Table 13.1 Suicide method in Canada (1997)

Hanging, strangulation and suffocation	39 per cent
Self-poisoning	26 per cent
Firearms	22 per cent
Jumping	4 per cent
Other	9 per cent

(Statistics Canada, 1997)

The role of primary care in detection and management of suicidality

Of people who complete suicide, 45 per cent have been seen by a primary care provider within the previous month. This figure is even higher in the elderly age group (Luoma et al., 2002).

Primary care providers can help prevent suicide by:
· identifying and treating depression aggressively
· monitoring for treatment-emergent suicidality in patients on antidepressant medications
· using antidepressants cautiously in adolescents
· following the American Psychiatric Association guidelines: seeing patients newly started on antidepressants weekly for four weeks, then every two weeks for four weeks, then at 12 weeks and as clinically indicated after 12 weeks (American Psychiatric Association Work Group on Suicidal Behaviors, 2003)
· flagging the charts of patients at higher risk of suicide
· closely monitoring patients at higher risk for suicide (see page 241):
  - patients with previous suicide attempts
  - patients with previous episodes of self-harm
  - patients recently discharged from psychiatric inpatient care
  - patients with a family history of suicide or suicide attempts
  - patients with a history of serious alcohol or other substance abuse
· using the powers of mental health legislation to intervene for protection.

Risk assessment is *not* suicide prediction

Because suicide is a relatively rare event, it is not possible to predict which individual will or will not attempt or complete suicide at any given point in time. *The clinician's job is to identify individuals at higher risk of suicide and take steps to lower that risk.*

Is your patient suicidal?

In clinical practice, concern about suicide risk begins with one or more of the following:

· recognition that a patient is seriously distressed or mentally unwell
· a clear or covert statement by the patient that he or she is considering suicide: *"I'm not sure how long I can go on like this." "I'm just so tired of being down."*
· communication from a family member or friend who is concerned about the patient: *"He keeps talking about how we'd be better off without him."*

ASK ABOUT SUICIDE
The clinician's responsibility is to investigate suicidal intent in the patient. The most direct, effective way to do this is to ask:
· "Have things gotten so bad that you've thought about hurting yourself or ending your life?"
· "Sometimes when people feel the way you do right now, they start to have thoughts about suicide. Has this ever happened to you?"

A calm, non-judgmental, concerned approach will tell the patient that you care, and that you will be able to cope with his or her answer.

Note: Asking about suicidal intent does not "plant" this as an idea in the patient.

Special situations:
· After a romantic relationship has ended, ask the patient whether he or she has thoughts about killing the former partner and/or children.
· In a female patient with postpartum depression and suicidality, ask about thoughts that the baby would be better off dead, intent to harm the child, and so on.

DO SCREENING QUESTIONNAIRES HELP?
Clinical assessment is the gold standard. Suicide screening instruments and scales:
· have unacceptably high false positive and false negative rates
· have poor generalizability
· have limited usefulness, functioning primarily as *aides mémoires* for the clinician.

INVESTIGATE THE SEVERITY OF THE SUICIDAL INTENT
If the patient endorses suicidal thoughts, the clinician's next task is to determine how serious the suicidal intent is.
Ask the patient:
· "What kinds of thoughts have you been having?" (This is a high-yield question so be sure to let the patient talk.)
· "How long have you been having these thoughts? When did they first start?"
· "How often are they happening? Daily? Weekly? All the time?"

Ask the patient to rate the severity of the suicidal thinking on a scale of 1 to 10, with 1 being very low intensity and 10 being extremely intense or severe.

Ask about a plan and access to means:
· "Do you have a plan for how you would kill yourself?"
· "Have you thought about any other methods?" (Patients may not reveal the most lethal method at first-ask.)
· "Do you have any firearms or other weapons at home? Where are they?"
· If the preferred method is overdose or hanging:
  - "Have you bought or saved pills? Do you have a rope?"
  - "Have you 'rehearsed' or 'gone through the motions' of killing yourself?"

Assess the patient's intent to act
"In the next 24–48 hours, how likely is it that you will act on your suicidal plan?" (Ask the patient to rate the likelihood on a scale of 1 to 10, with 1 being very unlikely and 10 being certain.)

Consider whether the patient has a history of impulsivity (high-risk behaviours, overspending, fights, poorly thought-out decisions). If you don't know the patient well, ask:
· "Would you consider yourself an impulsive person?"
· "Have you recently felt out of control at times?"

Self-harm versus suicidality
Not all patients who harm themselves by cutting, burning or other mutilating behaviours are actively suicidal.

To differentiate self-harm from suicidal behaviour, ask about the person's intentions. Was the cutting (burning, etc.) done to end the person's life, to gain relief from emotional distress, or to overcome a feeling of numbness?

Remember, patients who self-harm may have more than one intention for the behaviour, and self-harm is a risk factor for future suicide attempts. Co-existence of both behaviours is more the rule than the exception in border-line personality and other impulsive personality disorders.

Identify factors that increase risk substantially

IMPAIRED REALITY TESTING
- Psychosis
- Intoxication with alcohol or other drugs
  Note: Do not permit the intoxicated suicidal patient to go home. Transfer the patient to an emergency room (see page 245).

HOPELESSNESS
- Ask the patient: "Are you feeling hopeless?" or "Can you see things getting better for you?"

PREVIOUS ATTEMPTED SUICIDE
- The more lethal the method used, the higher the risk.
- The risk increases with each attempt.
- People who have had multiple suicide attempts should be considered chronically at risk.
- People who were recently discharged from an inpatient psychiatric ward, particularly if suicide was attempted, are at risk.

CURRENT SEVERE PSYCHIATRIC DISORDER
- Major depression
- Schizophrenia
- Alcohol abuse/dependence
- Borderline and antisocial personality disorders, especially in combination with major depression

OTHER FACTORS KNOWN TO INCREASE RISK
· Family history of suicide (there is likely a genetic as well as a family environment contribution)
· Alcohol abuse
· Debilitating medical illness
· Recent loss (divorce, unemployment, death of someone close)

Assess reasons for living and factors that may be protective

Ask the patient:
· "Things have been pretty rough. What keeps you going?"
· "You've been thinking about suicide, but you say you wouldn't follow through. What keeps you from harming yourself?"

Factors that may be associated with lower suicidal risk include:
· religious beliefs that suicide is wrong
· married state
· children under 18 years of age living at home
· employment
· strong therapeutic relationship
· good problem-solving skills
· generally higher level of self-esteem.

Management of the suicidal patient

All people who are suicidal are ambivalent, wanting to die and wanting to live. Keep in mind that suicidality is a fluid state and can change dramatically in the space of a few hours.

Management should focus on:
· optimizing the safety of the person
· communicating concern, caring and support
· intervening wherever possible to decrease risk and increase reasons for living
· providing immediate symptomatic relief for insomnia, agitation, anxiety.

Table 13.2 Management of suicidality issues for specific psychiatric diagnoses

PSYCHIATRIC DIAGNOSIS	IMPLICATIONS FOR MANAGEMENT
Major depressive disorder	Antidepressants can increase suicidality (uncommon); occurs early; may be higher in adolescents. Follow up weekly for first four weeks; biweekly for next four weeks.
Schizophrenia	Clozapine is indicated in patients at high risk for suicidal behaviour.
Bipolar disorder	Lithium may be the drug of choice in patients at high risk for suicidal behaviour.
Substance abuse/ dependence	Assess over early weeks of abstinence/decreased intake for sustained depression.
Borderline personality disorder	Dialectical behavioural therapy and other psychotherapies can reduce the risk of suicidal behaviour (see page 152).

· treating identified psychiatric disorders (see Table 13.2 for management of suicidality issues for specific psychiatric diagnoses)
· offering hope of a positive treatment outcome.

Personal safety for primary care providers is equally important. If a suicidal patient is threatening in any way, remove yourself and others from the situation and call 911.

Management of the patient with a suicide plan and high intent

If your patient has a plan and tells you that he or she has a strong intent to follow through, or if the plan is highly lethal (e.g., firearm), further questioning is probably not warranted. This patient should be transferred immediately to the nearest emergency room (see page 245).

Management of the patient with low intent but with serious risk factors

If your patient denies a plan, or has low intent to follow through in the short term, but has one or more serious risk factors, request an urgent psychiatric consultation (within 24 to 48 hours) and:

· Wherever possible (with the patient's agreement) get corroborative history from family, friends or co-workers to confirm your assessment of risk.
· Remove lethal weapons and medications from the home. Have a responsible family member or friend call you to report that this has been done. If you have reason to doubt that the weapons/medications have been removed, involve the police.
· Ensure that the patient and his or her family know how to reach you if suicidal thoughts worsen.
· Provide symptomatic relief (e.g., small quantities of benzodiazepine for agitation or insomnia; prescribe a high enough dose to be effective).
· See the patient the next day to reassess, and then frequently (as dictated by level of suicidal intent) until psychiatric consultation takes place.

Management of the patient with suicidal thoughts but no plan

Patients who have suicidal thoughts but no plan and *no serious risk factors* (e.g., previous attempt) can often be managed in the primary care setting.
· Talk to a family member, friend or co-worker of the patient to confirm your impressions and get additional history.
· Remove any lethal weapons or dangerous amounts of medication from the home. Have a responsible family member or friend call you to report that this has been done. If you have reason to doubt that the weapons/medications have been removed, check with another family member or involve the police if firearms are involved.
· Ensure that your patient and his or her family know how to reach you if suicidal thoughts worsen.
· If your patient lives alone, try to find a family member or friend who will stay with the person until treatment begins to have an effect.
· Provide symptomatic relief (e.g., small quantities of benzodiazepine for agitation or insomnia; prescribe a high enough dose for it to be effective).

· Start treatment for depression. Whenever possible use an SSRI in preference to more lethal drugs such as tricyclic medications or MAOIs. Educate your patient about depression and communicate hope and reassurance about a positive treatment outcome.
· Encourage the patient to reduce or eliminate the use of alcohol.
· Address relationship issues and other stressors — refer for counselling if you do not provide counselling yourself.
· See the patient at least weekly for the first month to monitor:
  - suicidality
  - compliance with treatment
  - side-effects of medication
  - response to treatment.

Transferring the high-risk patient for emergency psychiatric consultation

· Do not leave the patient alone.
· Place the patient in as safe an environment as is possible.
· Tell the patient you want him or her to be seen by a psychiatrist as soon as possible.
· Call for an urgent consultation.
· Give the emergency room physician or the on-call psychiatrist as much information as you can, including any history of psychiatric disorders, past suicide attempts, family history of suicide attempts, current stressors, current medical conditions and medications. Whenever possible send a brief note. For example:

> This 45-year-old male patient has a history of serious unipolar depression with one suicide attempt in the past. He is currently going through a difficult divorce, is depressed and expressing hopelessness, suicidal intent, with a plan to overdose on his antidepressants. He is medically well except for mild hypertension. His current medications are: hydrochlorothiazide 25 mg per day, and sertraline 150 mg per day.

· Have your staff call a family member or friend of the patient.

If the patient is co-operative and wants help

If the patient is co-operative, the person can be transferred to hospital as a voluntary patient with a responsible family member or friend. Some emergency rooms will expect you to have done a basic "medical clearance." This usually involves questioning the patient about drug ingestion, and doing vitals and a basic neurological examination.

Let the emergency room know when the patient leaves your office and when they should expect the patient to arrive. Ask to be called if the patient does not arrive within a reasonable time. If the patient does not arrive, call the patient's home. If you cannot locate the patient, call police and tell them your concerns, and ask them to apprehend and take the patient to the nearest emergency room. Familiarize yourself with your jurisdiction's mental health legislation to be able to use its powers appropriately to help your patients.

If the patient is not co-operative

If the patient refuses to go to the emergency room, tell the patient that you are very concerned and that you are obliged by law to ensure his or her safety. Call police and request that they take the patient to the nearest emergency room. Be prepared to give a description of the patient if he or she leaves your office. Do not try to *physically* stop the patient.

Community and online resources

- Suicide ... Read This First (www.metanoia.org/suicide). A useful website for people who are thinking about suicide. It offers hope, understanding, ways to cope with the emotional pain the person is experiencing, and a persuasive argument for delaying suicide and getting help.
- Canadian Association for Suicide Prevention (www.suicideprevention.ca). This site has a list of Canadian crisis centres with contact information, lists of related/supportive organizations and useful links to other good websites. See in particular *The CASP Blueprint for a Canadian National Suicide Prevention Strategy*.

- Befrienders (www.befrienders.org). A confidential 24-hour e-mail service for people in distress, run by the Samaritans. The site provides access to emotional support and the opportunity to "talk" to someone in 20 languages and provides a list of helplines (distress centres) by country and province/ state, with the phone number and e-mail address.
- Centre for Suicide Prevention (www.suicideinfo.ca). Provides excellent information about youth at risk of suicide for professionals working with young people and parents. The site outlines warning signs, how to communicate with a potentially suicidal young person, and how to take action before or after suicide. It also provides advice about the care of parents with a suicidal youth. The section for the suicidal youth is still under development.
- *Survivors of Suicide Handbook* (available at www.speak-out.ca). A handbook written by the families of individuals who died by suicide for survivors who have lost someone to suicide. It offers practical information about the legal aftermath of suicide, the grieving process and coping with the shock of suicide, how to talk about the suicide with friends and family, how to deal with financial issues and insurance, plus it provides a list of other resources that provide support, comfort and advice.

References

American Psychiatric Association Work Group on Suicidal Behaviors, Jacobs, D.G., Baldessarini, R.J., Conwell, Y., Fawcett, J.A., Horton, L., Meltzer, H. et al. (2003). Practice guideline for the assessment and treatment of patients with suicidal behaviors. *American Journal of Psychiatry, 160* (11 Suppl.), 1–60.

Canadian Association for Suicide Prevention. (2009). *The CASP Blueprint for a Canadian National Suicide Prevention Strategy* (2nd ed.). Winnipeg, MB: Canadian Association for Suicide Prevention.

Luoma, J.B., Martin, C.E. & Pearson, J.L. (2002). Contact with mental health and primary care providers before suicide: A review of the evidence. *American Journal of Psychiatry, 159* (6), 909–915.

Mann, J., Apter, A., Bertolote, J., Beautrais, A., Currier, D., Haas, A. et al. (2005). Suicide prevention strategies. A systematic review. *Journal of the American Medical Association, 294* (16), 2064–2074. DOI: 10.1001/jama.294.16.2064

Rudd, M.D. (2006). *The Assessment and Management of Suicidality.* Sarasota, FL: Professional Resource Press.

Sakinofsky, I. (Ed.). (2007). Caring for the suicidal patient: An evidence-based approach. *Canadian Journal of Psychiatry, 52* (6 Suppl.), 1S-136S.

Statistics Canada, Health Statistics Division. (1997). Mortality summary list of causes, 1997 (Cat. No. 84-209). Ottawa: Minister of Industry.

14
Psychotherapy in primary care

ARI E. ZARETSKY

Introduction

Many primary care providers avoid psychotherapy with their patients even when they identify and diagnose mood and anxiety disorders. They may perceive this treatment to be too difficult to learn, beyond the scope of their practice and too time-consuming to be cost-effective or feasible within a busy practice.

Unfortunately, because referral to a specialist such as a psychiatrist or psychologist is often associated with long delays, patients with psychiatric problems run the risk of not receiving comprehensive treatment if primary care providers refrain from using psychotherapy.

This chapter presents a model of psychotherapy for primary care providers that is pragmatic and brief and integrates strategies including cognitive-behavioural therapy (CBT), interpersonal therapy (IPT) and solution-focused psychotherapy.

Indications for primary care psychotherapy for mood and anxiety disorders

· Patient preference (either as an adjunct to, or alternative to, pharmacotherapy)
· Mild to moderate major depression (PHQ-9 score of 5–14)

· Dysthymic disorder
· Mild to moderate anxiety disorder
· Somatic complaints that appear to have a significant psychological component
  and the patient appears to have some insight

Pharmacotherapy and psychotherapy

Many patients' adherence to pharmacotherapy improves when they receive
psychotherapy. Patients who are sensitive to medication side-effects or concerned with long-term safety of antidepressant medication may prefer psychotherapy. Patients who wish to taper off antidepressants before becoming
pregnant may also prefer psychotherapy. Similarly, patients who are already
pregnant and who would like to come off medication may want to pursue
psychotherapy.

Psychotherapy and severe depression

Patients with severe depression should only receive psychotherapy as
an adjunct rather than a primary treatment. The efficacy of psychotherapy
for severe depression is controversial and appears to be highly dependent
on the skill of the psychotherapist. Psychotherapy can be provided as
an adjunct for severe depression but should never compromise or delay
optimal pharmacotherapy. Ongoing close evaluation of the patient's clinical
status and referral to an expert psychologist or psychiatrist is indicated when
the patient fails to improve or suicidal potential escalates.

Psychotherapy and chronic depression, bipolar disorder and somatoform disorders

Some simple psychotherapy strategies can be integrated into the treatment
of bipolar disorder. Chronic depression, although difficult to treat with
psychotherapy alone, can benefit from a combination of antidepressant
medication and psychotherapy. Common conditions seen by primary care
providers such as somatoform disorders (e.g., pain disorder associated
with psychological factors or hypochondriasis) can sometimes be treated
effectively using CBT strategies.

Contraindications to psychotherapy in primary care

· Psychosis (e.g., psychotic depression, mania, schizophrenia)
· Organic mental disorder (e.g., dementia)
· Antisocial personality disorder and severe borderline personality disorders
· Severe substance abuse/dependence
· Poor psychological insight

Although promising evidence-based psychotherapy treatment interventions based on specific manuals have been developed for schizophrenia and bipolar disorder, these approaches are too sub-specialized for most primary care providers.

Personality disorders are not a contraindication for psychotherapy in primary care given that treatments like CBT for depression do not appear to be consistently negatively affected by comorbid personality disorder. However, disruptive personality disorders like antisocial personality disorder or borderline personality disorder are far more difficult to treat and qualified expertise is strongly advised in order to avert boundary violations.

Patients with eating disorders, obsessive-compulsive disorder (OCD) and posttraumatic stress disorder (PTSD) can be effectively treated by CBT. However, the treatment approach is quite sub-specialized and requires extensive expertise that is beyond the scope of family medicine. Supportive psychotherapy is indicated and referral to a mental health practitioner with expertise in these areas is indicated.

Although moderate substance use is not an absolute contraindication for adjunctive psychotherapy, psychotherapy provided by a primary care provider should never compromise or delay treatment for severe substance abuse/dependence.

Any significant impairment in cognition (from any cause) will also make psychotherapy very difficult to deliver effectively. Careful assessment of the patient's capacity to read and comprehend is extremely important.

Somatoform conditions, especially when the patient has very poor insight, are extremely difficult to treat psychotherapeutically and are usually beyond the scope of expertise of a primary care provider.

Models of short-term psychotherapy for primary care

Cognitive-behavioural therapy (CBT)
· A here-and-now active therapeutic collaboration that examines underlying assumptions/beliefs, challenges them and tests them out
· Based on a cognitive model (thoughts and behaviour determine emotional reactions to stressful life events)
· Structured (agenda is set and followed each session)
· Goal-oriented (behavioural goals are delineated and measured throughout therapy)
· Time-limited (typically 12 sessions for anxiety; 16 to 20 sessions for depression)
· Based on a teaching model (goal is to teach the patient skills to become his or her own therapist)
· Includes homework assignments to enhance skill acquisition (often using self-help manuals)
· Teaches relapse prevention

Interpersonal therapy (IPT)
· Based on psychodynamic and interpersonal models (psychological problems are due to communication problems, which are formed due to insecure attachment styles and early life experiences)
· Recognizes roles of genetic, neurobiological, developmental and personality factors as predisposing and precipitating factors for depression
· Views depression as a medical illness that occurs within a social context: interpersonal issues are linked to depressed mood and depression impairs interpersonal functioning
· Focuses on the interpersonal factors that perpetuate depression
· Assesses the patient's past history in a detailed manner

- Assists patients to communicate their interpersonal needs and emotions more effectively
- Provides comprehensive psychoeducation about depression (including ways that the patient has adopted the "sick role" of depression)
- Identifies one to two focal areas for time-limited therapeutic work: interpersonal disputes, role transitions, bereavement, interpersonal deficits
- Typically consists of 16 weekly sessions

Solution-focused therapy (SFT)

- Pragmatic, active therapy that emphasizes a specific therapeutic style/stance rather than specific techniques and theories of psychopathology
- Based on social constructionist philosophy
- More creative, flexible and less "manualized" than CBT and IPT
- Style can be integrated into CBT and IPT
- Focuses on what patients want to achieve through therapy rather than on the problems that made them seek help
- Does not focus on the past but on the present and future
- Encourages the patient to create a concrete vision of a "preferred future" and then pay attention to any movement toward this image
- Focuses on the patient's "personal story," his or her strengths and resources
- Carefully studies exceptions to the patient's problem (when the problems are not as severe).

Committing time for psychotherapy

Long-term psychotherapy, although commonly practised in the community, is not recommended for patients with currently active Axis I mood or anxiety disorders.

CBT, IPT and SFT all require the clinician to be very comfortable using general supportive psychotherapy techniques of active listening, empathy, warmth and genuineness. In addition, CBT, IPT and SFT will also require the allocation of time to initially meet with the patient on a regular basis rather than scheduling sessions as needed.

Although sessions need not be scheduled for 45–50 minutes, a minimum of 16–30 minutes once a week is necessary in order to develop rapport and create sufficient momentum to achieve therapeutic success.

What form of psychotherapy works best in primary care?

· There are few overall efficacy differences between CBT and IPT for mild to moderate depression.
· CBT is the most comprehensively studied psychotherapy and is the first choice for anxiety disorders. (There is currently only weak evidence for the efficacy of IPT in anxiety disorders.)
· CBT may be used alone for anxiety disorders, particularly if the condition is mild.
· CBT has a broad spectrum of action beyond mood and anxiety disorders (efficacy demonstrated for eating disorders, substance abuse, chronic fatigue, sexual dysfunction, anger control, etc.).
· SFT has not been studied as systematically but appears to be effective in mild depression.
· CBT has some advantages over IPT: less psychotherapy experience is required by the therapist, the structure is beneficial for more symptomatic patients and there is extensive availability of supplementary self-help bibliotherapy such as *Mind Over Mood* or the *The Feeling Good Handbook* (see the resources at the end of this chapter).
· IPT has some advantages over CBT: less emphasis on formal homework, writing and language skills and structure; evidence of efficacy in non-Western populations and patients from lower socioeconomic backgrounds.

Integrating psychotherapy in primary care

The recommended approach for primary care providers doing psychotherapy is to integrate strategies from CBT, IPT and SFT. This "modified CBT-lite" approach is pragmatic, highly active and supportive; emphasizes addressing one or two core problems in the here and now; and leverages and reinforces the patient's own inner strengths to achieve change. Momentum is created by consistently adopting a therapeutically optimistic stance, refraining from excessive focus on the patient's past or the patient's psychopathology. Psychoeducation about mental illness (usually including family members) is also an integral component of this treatment as is bibliotherapy and self-help exercises.

Adjunctive psychotherapy for depression and anxiety

Case scenario

The case that follows is intended to provide a practical illustration of when psychotherapy could be usefully integrated into a primary care setting.

Ms. A. made an appointment to see her primary care physician because she had not been feeling well for the past six months. In addition to her episodic tearfulness and five kilogram weight loss, Ms. A. told her physician that she had lost pleasure in most of her day-to-day activities and that she had very little energy during the day. Her inability to concentrate at work and her constant irritability, self-criticism, guilt and pessimism were other issues that she raised with her primary care physician. Ms. A. also reported that she frequently worried about things, and that the worry was almost impossible to control. Over the last six months Ms. A. had also experienced at least one full-blown panic attack a week with tachypnea, hyperventilation, dyspnea, lightheadedness and a feeling of intense dread. This had resulted in a progressive restriction of her life such that she was avoiding using public transit and was avoiding using elevators as well as shopping malls. Finally, Ms. A. also described difficulty sleeping through the night, which was puzzling to her since she was often tired and lethargic during the day.

Ms. A. is a lawyer with three young children. Her husband is frequently away on business, which is an enduring source of resentment and conflict in the marriage. In addition, Ms. A.'s father died exactly one year before the onset of depressive symptoms and at the time of his death, Ms. A. had not had the time to attend the funeral in a distant city due to pressing child care and work obligations. Ms. A. had a conflicted relationship with her father, whom she experienced as harsh, demanding and critical. Ms. A. herself was a perfectionist with harsh, unrelenting standards.

Ms. A.'s primary care physician listened carefully to the history during the 15-minute appointment. She carefully evaluated the risk for suicide and dangerousness to others and ruled these both out as clinical concerns. She then did a brief medical assessment including testing to rule out anemia and hypothyroidism. Ms. A.'s physician was aware of a family history of clinical depression and suspected that major depression and panic disorder with agoraphobia were the most likely diagnoses. The primary care physician prescribed the SSRI escitalopram.

Four weeks later, during a follow-up appointment, Ms. A. reported feeling better, as some of her symptoms had improved. Ms. A.'s primary care physician was glad that the prescribed SSRI medication appeared to be working. She booked a number of brief follow-up appointments with Ms. A. lasting 10 minutes each over the next two months focusing primarily on assessing symptoms of depression and anxiety as well as medication adherence and side-effects. The primary care physician then suggested that Ms. A. could come back in six months.

Four months later, the symptoms of depression had resurfaced. Ms. A. was initially reluctant to return to her primary care physician because she was frustrated with the treatment and had begun to lose hope that she would ever feel better. She began to have thoughts such as: "maybe this is just me and I just have to accept it." Ms. A. eventually did present to her family physician but complained primarily about her poor sleep, her loss of appetite and her poor energy rather than depression or life issues.

Phase I: Medicalize and psychologize the psychiatric illness (sessions 1 – 2)

The primary care provider should take an in-depth history to identify psychosocial precipitants of the depressive relapse (e.g., losses, role transitions, interpersonal disputes). After identifying precipitants, the primary care provider should ask:

- "How have these events affected your view of yourself, the world and the future?"
- "Are these negative views that you have new or have you carried them for a long time?"
- "If you have carried these views for a long time, where did you learn these beliefs?"

The clinician should provide psychoeducation about depression and anxiety (in this case the anxiety disorder is panic disorder with agoraphobia). Invite family members to attend the psychoeducation session. Present these disorders as treatable and reversible medical conditions that have profound psychological and interpersonal manifestations. Reading material should be provided as well as appropriate websites (see the list of resources, page 262).

The primary care provider should emphasize a broad treatment approach that combines pharmacotherapy with psychotherapy. Discuss the rationale for combining pharmacotherapy with psychotherapy, including:

- more comprehensive treatment of psychosocial problems with psychotherapy
- faster resolution of symptoms with pharmacotherapy
- better overall outcome with combination
- better adherence to medication with psychotherapy
- relapse prevention with psychotherapy.

Explicitly address stigma and provide a more balanced alternative to the patient's self-critical thinking (e.g., "I am defective"):

- "Many patients with depression or anxiety have difficulty accepting their conditions and have negative thoughts. What goes through your mind when you think about your problems with depression and anxiety?"

Examine thoughts that may interfere with medication adherence:
· "The last time you forgot to take your medication, what went through your mind?"

Make a list of the advantages and disadvantages of taking medication from the patient's perspective and then try to address the disadvantages.

Thoughts

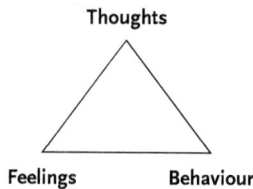

Feelings   **Behaviour**

Socialize the patient to the cognitive model. Draw a triangle with thoughts, feelings and behaviour at the three points. Use any situation where there is a negative mood shift and ask the patient if he or she can identify thoughts, feelings and behaviours (internal physical reactions or external overt behaviour). After dissecting a problematic situation (e.g., non-adherence with medication, feelings of shame about diagnosis), write down the patient's thoughts, feelings and behaviour on the three points of the triangle. Ask the patient if the cognitive model has any relevance to him or her in dealing with his or her current problems. If the patient can readily identify thoughts and recognize their importance within the first session, this suggests that cognitive interventions such as cognitive restructuring will be feasible. If the patient does not fully comprehend the relevance of the cognitive model, consider emphasizing behavioural activation, exposure strategies and problem-solving approaches in psychotherapy.
· Contract for a 12- to-16-session course of psychotherapy.
· Ask the patient to commit in writing to doing self-help reading and writing exercises for one to two hours between therapy sessions. Explain the rationale for writing things down in a log.
· Have the patient write down a "problem list" in the first session and from this problem list generate two to three specific behavioural goals for therapy.

At least one of these goals should be interpersonal in nature (e.g., addressing a conflict with another person).

· As homework after the first session, ask the patient to create a concrete vision of his or her preferred future.

Phase II: Gather more information about dysfunctional behaviour, thoughts and interpersonal problems (sessions 3 – 5)

· Measure symptoms of depression with the PHQ-9 or Beck Depression Inventory II (BDI-II).
· Try to meet twice a week (for 15 – 30 minutes per session) over the first month of treatment to create momentum.
· Set an agenda and follow the general structure of CBT sessions outlined in Table 14.1 on page 260.
· Always review homework assignments early in the session.
· Regularly address medication adherence and medication side-effects at the beginning of each session for not more than five minutes.
· Assign the patient chapters to read on overcoming depression and anxiety in the *Mind Over Mood* workbook.
· If the patient is able to understand the cognitive model, assign chapters 1 – 5 from the *Mind Over Mood* workbook. Ask the patient to track negative automatic thoughts by filling out the first three columns of the automatic thought record.
· If lethargy is a major problem, begin behavioural activation by assigning two activities for the patient to do per day and have the patient record these activities on a log for you to review for the next two to four weeks.
· If anxiety and avoidance is a major problem, teach controlled breathing in the session and assign for homework. Ask the patient to create a hierarchy of feared situations that he or she is avoiding day-to-day.
· Assess the patient's interpersonal relationships by asking the patient to create an inventory of all significant past and current relationships, the current frequency of contact and the current quality of these relationships.

Table 14.1 Recommended structure for CBT sessions

1. Set an agenda, asking patients what they want to cover today.

2. Ask for feedback on the previous session—what they recall, what was useful, what bothered them, etc.

3. Check mood using the Beck Depression Inventory II.

4. Review homework and what was learned; address thoughts interfering with adherence.

5. Address new issues on agenda.

6. Ask the patient to summarize the session and collaboratively set new homework.

7. Request feedback.

Phase III: Begin cognitive restructuring and focused behavioural interventions (sessions 6–12)

· Continue to track mood (with PHQ-9 or BDI-II), feedback from sessions and medication adherence.

· Assign the automatic thought record and chapters 6–7 from the *Mind Over Mood* workbook.

· For anxiety, begin graded exposure assignments using the previously developed fear hierarchy of the patient as a guide.

· Address two salient interpersonal issues (e.g., loss, role transition, conflict, interpersonal deficits).

· If unassertiveness is a significant problem, teach interpersonal effectiveness via role playing. Also assign chapters pertaining to communication skills (chapters 18–22) from *The Feeling Good Handbook*. Also, the chapter on behavioural experiments from *Mind Over Mood* (chapter 8) can be assigned.

· Consider one or two couple sessions if marital stress is a major complicating factor and the patient and his or her partner agree to participate.

- If the patient is psychologically minded and capable of reflecting on deeper patterns of behaviour revealed in his or her automatic thought records, assign chapters on assumptions and core beliefs and guilt and shame (chapters 9 and 12) from *Mind Over Mood*.
- For deeper reflection on enduring dysfunctional personality patterns (e.g., perfectionism, interpersonal submissiveness, excessive mistrust, etc.) assign *Reinventing Your Life*.

Phase IV: Relapse prevention and termination (sessions 12–16)

- Continue to track mood (with PHQ-9 or BDI-II), feedback and medication adherence.
- Attribute improvement to the patient's actions rather than medication alone.
- Review what problems brought the patient into treatment, future scenarios that could precipitate relapse, what the patient learned to cope with mood/anxiety problems, what the patient needs to keep practising.
- Consider assigning meditation as a relapse prevention strategy. Assign reading and listening to a meditation CD from *The Mindful Way Through Depression*.
- Provide the patient with booster sessions (monthly tapered to bimonthly over the course of one year).

What psychotherapy is reasonable to expect from a primary care clinician

- Diagnose Axis I mood and anxiety disorder and develop a biopsychosocial treatment plan.
- Use behavioural activation strategies for lethargic patients with depression.
- Generate simple exposure hierarchies for patients with panic disorder and patients with phobic avoidance.
- Assign pertinent self-help bibliotherapy for uncomplicated depression and anxiety.

When to refer to a specialist

· Complicating comorbidity (significant substance abuse/dependence, severe personality disorder, complex anxiety disorder such as PTSD, OCD), severe eating disorder
· Severe presentation (serious suicidality, psychosis, bipolar disorder [especially Bipolar I, with manic episodes])
· Refractory to 12–16 sessions of combined treatment with medication and pharmacotherapy
· Concern about maintaining professional boundaries with patient

Community and online resources

Medical supports

· Community mental health clinics or hospital-based psychiatry outpatient clinics
· University- or hospital-affiliated cognitive therapy and interpersonal therapy clinics

Self-help or support groups

· Canadian Mental Health Association: www.cmha.ca
· Local mood disorders support groups, see Mood Disorders Society of Canada: www.mooddisorderscanada.ca

Self-management resources

· *The Feeling Good Handbook* by Dr. David D. Burns, Penguin Books, 1999.
· *Mind Over Mood* by David Greenberg and Christine Padesky, Guilford Press, 1995.
· *Reinventing Your Life: How to Break Free of Negative Life Patterns* by Jeffrey Young and Janet Klosko, Penguin Books, 1993.
· *The Mindful Way Through Depression* by Mark Williams, John Teasedale, Zindel Segal and Jon Kabat-Zinn, Guilford Press, 2007.

Online resources

- Internet Mental Health: www.internetmentalhealth.com
- Canadian Network for Mood and Anxiety Treatments: www.canmat.org
- Canadian Mental Health Association: www.cmha.ca
- Mood Disorders Society of Canada: www.mooddisorderscanada.ca
- National Institute of Mental Health: www.nimh.nih.gov
- Academy of Cognitive Therapy: www.academyofcognitivetherapy.org
- British Association for Behavioural and Cognitive Psychotherapies: www.babcp.com
- Centre for Addiction and Mental Health: www.camh.net.

References

Butler, A.C., Chapman, J.E., Forman, E.M. & Beck, A.T. (2006). The empirical status of cognitive-behavioral therapy: A review of meta-analyses. *Clinical Psychology Review, 26* (1), 17–31. DOI: 10.1016/j.cpr.2005.07.003

DeRubies, R.J., Hollon, S.D., Amsterdam, J.D., Shelton, R.C., Young, P.R., Salomon, R. et al. (2005). Cognitive therapy vs medications in the treatment of moderate to severe depression. *Archives of General Psychiatry, 62* (4), 409–416.

Fiejo de Mello, M., de Jesus Mari, J., Bacaltchuk, J., Verdeli, H. & Neugebauer, R. (2005). A systematic review of research findings on the efficacy of interpersonal therapy for depressive disorders. *European Archives of Psychiatry and Clinical Neuroscience, 255* (2), 74–82. DOI: 10.1007/s00406-004-0542-x

Gingerich, W.J. & Eisengart, S. (2000). Solution-focused brief therapy: A review of the outcome research. *Family Process, 39* (4), 477–498. DOI: 10.1111/j.1545-5300.2000.39408.x

Hollon, S.D., DeRubies, R.J., Shelton, R.C., Amsterdam, J.D., Salomon, R.M., O'Reardin, J.P. et al. (2005). Prevention of relapse following cognitive therapy vs medications in moderate to severe depression. *Archives of General Psychiatry, 62* (4), 417–422.

King, M., Davidson, O., Taylor, F., Haines, A., Sharp, D., & Turner, R. (2002). Effectiveness of teaching general practitioners skills in brief cognitive behaviour therapy to treat patients with depression: Randomized controlled trial. *British Medical Journal, 324* (7343), 947. DOI: 10.1136/bmj.324.7343.947

Klomek, A.B. & Mufson, L. (2006). Interpersonal psychotherapy for depressed adolescents. *Child & Adolescent Psychiatric Clinics of North America, 15* (4), 959–975.

Maccarelli, L. (2002). Maintenance interpersonal psychotherapy (IPT-M) treatment specificity: The impact on length of remission in women with recurrent depression. *Dissertation Abstracts International: Section B: The Sciences and Engineering, 63,* 536.

Rollman, B.L., Benlap, B.H., Reynolds, C.F., Schulberg, H.C. & Shear, M.K. (2003). A contemporary protocol to assist primary care physicians in the treatment of panic and generalized anxiety disorders. *General Hospital Psychiatry, 25,* 74–82.

Stein, M.B., Sherbourne, C.D., Craske, M.G., Means-Christensen, A., Bystritisky, A., Katon, W. et al. (2004). Quality of care for primary care patients with anxiety disorders. *American Journal of Psychiatry, 161* (12), 2230–2237.

Teasdale, J.D., Fennell, M.J., Hibbert, G.A. & Amies, P.L. (1984). Cognitive therapy for major depressive disorder in primary care. *British Journal of Psychiatry, 144* (4), 400–406.

Van Schaik, A., van Marwijk, H., Ader, H., van Dyck, R., de Haan, M., Penninx, B. et al. (2006). Interpersonal psychotherapy for elderly patients in primary care. *American Journal of Geriatric Psychiatry, 14* (9), 777–786.

15
Disability and insurance claims in primary care

ASH BENDER

Introduction

Mental health claims are now the largest category of short- and long-term disability cases and have become a routine part of any clinical practice. Mental disorders are now frequently cited as the most disabling illness affecting working individuals aged 18 to 44 in Western nations (Murray & Lopez, 1997). Unfortunately, disability-related issues can be one of the most challenging and time-consuming components of your practice, but they are critical to your patients given that the negative aspects of disability include:

· financial loss
· loss of occupational identity
· stigma and social isolation
· diminished future occupational and economic attainment
· higher rates of medical and mental disorders
· dependency on what can be an adversarial insurance or public social support system.

Included in this chapter are some practical guidelines for addressing mental health disability from your office with the goal of promoting recovery and return to work.

Key definitions

IMPAIRMENT

Impairment refers to problems with body function or structure such
as a significant deviation or loss (WHO, 2001).

DISABILITY

Disability refers to health-related restriction or lack of ability to perform
any activity, within a range considered normal (WHO, 1980).

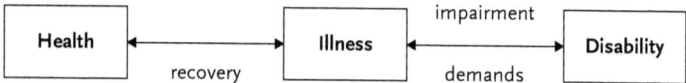

As a rule, total disability occurs only when demands cannot be modified
sufficiently to accommodate the impairment due to a mental health problem.

Documentation

All insurers, including government-sponsored workers' compensation
programs, require medical documentation in order to support a mental
health disability claim. Although documentation can be onerous, failure to
complete documents properly will result in significant distress and financial
burden to your patient. More recently, physicians have been found liable
for failure to provide documentation in a timely and complete manner.
Physicians are not required to provide medical information directly to
employers and should only do so after obtaining consent (Demeter &
Andersson, 2003).

· Complete forms in a timely and legible manner. If the forms are not
  completed, your patient will not receive benefits.
· Document when symptoms first appeared as payments may be made
  retroactively.
· List all supporting symptoms for the most responsible diagnosis.
· Use DSM diagnostic criteria only.

· Provide recommended treatment plan with return to work as a goal.
· Recommend any further investigations or treatment you cannot provide.
· Clearly note why the individual is impaired.
· Recommend clear work restrictions to assist accommodation by the employer.
· Recommend total disability as a last resort.

Compensation

Most occupation-related medical services and forms are not covered under provincial insurance plans and require separate billing. In such cases the physician should submit an invoice with a request for reasonable compensation (Ontario Medical Association, 2007). Most government-based requests have fixed fees that are clearly identified on the forms.

Insurance companies or lawyers may not provide information related to fees, and it is suggested that a fee be agreed upon before proceeding. Rates for these services are typically higher than government-funded remuneration. Regulatory bodies and medical associations can provide guidelines for billing.

Examples of services to third-party providers that would be billed for include:
· preparation of documents and transfer of files
· telephone calls or consultations for insurance companies
· insurance certificates and reports
· medical examinations or procedures for licensing or insurance
· Canada Pension Plan and Workers' Compensation reports.

Claim-related questions by insurers

Insurers request documented information to determine eligibility and extent of coverage required based on degree of disability. The information may be requested by an adjudicator, who manages terms and costs, and/or the case manager, who oversees treatment.

Below is a typical set of questions that will be elaborated on throughout this chapter (Dorian & Bender, 2010).

Cause
Is this a work-related psychological injury?

Onset
When did the symptoms first arise?

Contributing factors
What other factors are contributing to the disability?

Pre-existing conditions
Is there evidence of pre-existing mental health impairment?

Diagnosis
What is the most fitting DSM diagnosis?

Capacity
Is the individual able to work in any capacity?
If yes, are restrictions required?
If no, what are the reasons?

Treatment
What is the proposed treatment plan?
Who is the treatment provider?
How long will it be required?

Prognosis

When is return to work expected?
What is the individual's prognosis for returning to work in his or her previous or modified position?

Documenting cause

The key question is, "*Is this a work-related psychological injury?*"

Cause is most important for claims covered by the workers' compensation system or by an automobile insurance provider. In these cases insurers have an obligation to the claimant if the identified impairment is the result of a workplace incident or an automobile accident.

For private insurance provided by employers, cause may be of no significance as they still have an obligation to replace lost wages due to disability.

EXAMPLES OF CAUSES OF MENTAL HEALTH DISABILITY
Workplace injury:
· anxiety
· depression
· chronic pain
· cognitive problems.
  Personal loss:
· depression.

Accepted causes including "stress" are expanding but not universally recognized. The workplace is typically not accepted as a cause of psychosis, mania or substance abuse/dependence, but may be identified as a precipitant or as contributing to the disability.

An exception would be if the symptoms arose following exposure to a toxin in the workplace (e.g., second-hand smoke).

MALINGERING

Due to the potential for financial gain, insurance claims are often treated with a degree of suspicion. Malingering by symptom exaggeration or intentional feigning must also be considered (American Psychiatric Association, 2000).

Key points about malingering

Malingering is involved in only 10 to 20 per cent of claims. Risk factors for malingering include:
· antisocial personality disorder
· inconsistent symptoms
· inconsistency between work and home functioning
· obvious financial gain.

Documenting onset

The key question is, *"When did the symptoms first arise?"*

First onset of symptoms, as documented in clinical records, is often used to determine cause. In general, the onset of symptoms is expected within six months of an identified occupational cause. This highlights the importance of screening for mental health problems during a disability claim of any kind. Failure to recognize symptoms will result in delayed entitlement or denial of access to specialized mental health treatment.

Documenting contributing factors

The key question is, *"What other factors are contributing to the disability?"*

Contributing factors are important for recognizing the multi-factorial nature of disability. Minor contributing factors do not usually affect entitlement but should be considered in treatment planning and prognosis including, for example:
· financial strain
· family problems
· conflict with employer
· concurrent medical problems.

Documenting pre-existing conditions

The key question is, "*Is there evidence of pre-existing mental health impairment?*"

If symptoms were pre-existing, it is important to clearly identify onset and degree of work impairment. For example, an individual with a major depressive disorder may have had no symptoms or mild symptoms that were successfully treated without impairing the person's ability to work. In contrast, an individual may have been frequently absent from work before becoming totally disabled following a workplace incident.

If mental health problems were present, always note symptom severity and degree of work impairment.

Documenting a diagnosis

The key question is, "*What is the most fitting DSM diagnosis?*"

SYMPTOMS AND FUNCTIONING

Physicians are trained to identify symptoms within a clinical setting and obtain a diagnosis. Currently, the insurance system in Canada uses the DSM-IV multi-axial system as the standard. This requires the physician to provide supporting symptoms for each diagnosis including Axis V, the Global Assessment of Functioning (GAF). Individuals experiencing total mental health disability are expected to have a GAF score of 50 or lower, or severe impairment.

Assessing functioning is critical for determining if a symptom is resulting in functional problems. See Table 15.1 for examples of DSM symptoms and possible corresponding areas of problematic workplace and interpersonal functioning.

A specific diagnosis may affect an individual differently, depending on the type of symptoms and specific job duties. Here are some examples:
· Major Depressive Disorder
  - fatigue

- cognitive problems
- uncontrollable crying
· Panic Disorder
  - preoccupation with health status
  - agoraphobia
· Posttraumatic Stress Disorder
  - triggered anxiety and anger
  - avoidance of trauma reminders.

It is important to note that total disability only arises when duties cannot be modified to meet the impairment due to the mental health problem.

Documenting capacity

The key questions are:
· *"Is the individual able to work in any capacity?"*
· *"If yes, are restrictions required?"*
· *"If no, what are the reasons?"*

TAKING A FUNCTIONAL HISTORY

Asking about functioning will clarify the diagnosis and help in assessing the current level of functioning and capacity to work. Below are a few straight-forward questions.

WORK FUNCTIONING

A key question to ask when determining functioning in the workplace is, *"What do you do in a typical day?"*

When inquiring about the nature of the person's work, be sure to determine:
· physical demands
· psychological demands
· responsibilities
· ability to work safely
· individual or team work
· relations with customers, co-workers and employer
· shift schedule
· travel requirements.

Table 15.1 Assessing functioning

SYMPTOM	FUNCTIONING
Irritability	Conflict
Sadness	Isolation
Anxiety	Avoidance
Anhedonia	Absenteeism
Helplessness	Poor motivation
Delusions	Engagement in relationships
	Inappropriate behaviour
Concentration	Work accuracy
Memory	Work efficiency
Executive function	Decision making
Sleep	Activities of daily living (ADLs)
	Household activities
Energy	Sexual activity
Psychomotor	Task vigilance
Pain	Violence and accidents
Intoxication	Coping behaviour

Such specific inquiries about the nature of the person's work are very important and are often missed. This will also strengthen recommendations for restrictions and suggested accommodation.

If suitable duties are not available or if the impairment is too severe, then total disability results.

Table 15.2 Taking a functional history

DOMAIN OF FUNCTIONING	QUESTION
ADLs	Are you caring for yourself as usual?
Instrumental ADLs	What activities do you do at home?
Hobbies	What do you do for pleasure?
Social	How is your social life?
Family	What do you do with your children?
Relationships	How are you getting along with your partner?
Sex	How is your sex life?
Work	Any problems at work? Any missed time?

Planning and documenting treatment

The key questions are:
- "What is the treatment plan?"
- "Who is the treatment provider?"
- "How long will treatment be required?"

PLANNING TREATMENT

Planning for a return to work should begin early and remain rehabilitation-focused. Ideally, both treatment and planning for a return to work would be done concurrently provided there are no barriers. Roles for primary care providers in planning treatment include:
- educating your patient about diagnosis, treatments and recovery
- identifying potential barriers to recovery
- clarifying duties and workplace supports
- discussing return to work from the beginning
- encouraging active coping
- asking the insurer about additional rehabilitation resources
- referring early for severe symptoms or total disability.

TIPS FOR YOUR PATIENT AT HOME
Drawing on behavioural activation, encourage "healthy" activity in order
to limit adaptation to the "sick role." Patients should be encouraged to:
· maintain self-care and family routine
· engage in cardiovascular exercise at least three times per week
· engage in activity scheduling with support network
· participate in physiotherapy for strength and pain
· maintain good sleep hygiene to keep routines
· pursue pleasurable activities.

THE ROLE OF SPECIALISTS WITHIN TREATMENT
Insurers will often cover fees for private providers such as psychologists
or occupational therapists as part of a treatment plan. Specialty services
are essential to mental health rehabilitation if disability becomes prolonged
(over 90 days). Note that it is important to choose capable and qualified
specialists who will be able to both focus treatment on return to work as
a goal and provide completed documentation.

The primary care provider may use specialist services when working with
the patient to:
· discourage passive coping such as "relaxing"
· access evidence-based treatments rather than "counselling."

Examples of services that specialists can provide in disability cases are
provided below.

Psychologist
· Cognitive-behavioural therapy (CBT)
· Interpersonal therapy (IPT)

Occupational therapist
· Behavioural activation
· Exposure-based therapy

Psychiatrist
- Confirmation of diagnosis
- Establishment of degree of impairment
- Stabilization of severe symptoms
- Recommendation on work restrictions
- Follow-up following return to work

EXAMPLES OF REHABILITATION-FOCUSED TREATMENTS
Cognitive
- Provide education regarding diagnosis and treatment.
- Set expectation for a full recovery.
- Identify perceived barriers to recovery.

Behavioural
- Encourage adaptive lifestyle modifications including:
  - improving sleep hygiene
  - limiting use of alcohol and other drugs
  - maintaining a schedule of activities when not working.

Medical
- Select medications for efficacy and side-effect profile:
  - NSAIDs for pain instead of narcotics
  - non-benzodiazepine sleep agents
  - antidepressants rather than benzodiazepines, when appropriate.
- Refer to appropriate specialists (psychology, occupational therapy, psychiatry) if recovery is delayed.

Returning to work

Patient readiness for return to work is the key factor. Asking about the positives and negatives about returning to work, with a focus on barriers, is a good approach (Franche & Krause, 2002). It is important to ask the patient:

· Is there anything good about going back to work?
· What are you afraid of? What may happen if you return to work?
· Do you foresee any barriers?

If suitably accommodated work is not available then retraining or rehabilitation to re-enter the workforce is an option. Direct inquiry with the
patient, insurer and employer is suggested if return-to-work supports
are not apparent.

Several programs exist that can assist financially or provide specialized
services:
· not-for-profit employment agencies
  - skills development programs
  - job searches
· federally funded programs
  - Canada Pension Plan
· provincially funded programs
  - Workers' Compensation
  - Employment Insurance
  - social assistance
  - disability support programs
· insurance-funded programs
  - return-to-work co-ordination
  - driving desensitization
  - work hardening
· employer-based programs
  - employee assistance programs
  - human resources.

COMMON BARRIERS TO RETURNING TO WORK
· Treatment adherence
· Medication side-effects
· Comorbidities
· Stigma

· Excessive demands
· Lack of home and employer supports
· Outstanding claim disputes
· Travel limitations

STEPS TOWARD A RETURN TO WORK
Preparing for return to work
· Understand the patient's current work position, including:
  - physical and psychological demands
  - responsibilities
  - current conflict
  - safety
  - management support.
· Carefully consider if suitable work accommodation is available
  and length of time needed:
  - hours (e.g., four hours/day for one month due to fatigue)
  - frequency
  - shifts
  - duties (e.g., no machine operation due to poor concentration)
  - transfer to different site.
· Enquire if additional supports are available at the workplace:
  - human resources
  - employee assistance programs
  - insurance coverage for medications/psychotherapy.
· Mediate to address disputed terms or grievances.

Initiating the process of returning to work
Your patient's successful return to work should procede along
the following sequence:
· Referral to return-to-work co-ordinator
· Onsite job visit by affected employee
· Gradual return to the workplace
· Gradual increase in hours or responsibilities
· Retraining if accommodated work is unavailable.

Helping your patient stay in the workplace
· Regularly monitor for symptoms and side-effects.
· Enhance problem-solving skills.
· Encourage active coping.

Communicating with employers

Managing mental health information with an employer is critical. Physicians are not required to communicate confidential health information to the employer unless they have specific consent. Only direct and clear information regarding the type and duration (temporary or permanent) of medical restrictions is required. Understanding employer-related issues will promote a successful return to work, though few workplaces have dedicated programs.

EMPLOYER'S PERSPECTIVES
Employers have inconsistent policies and procedures addressing a return to work following mental health disability. Unfortunately, few have established return-to-work programs (Canadian Psychiatric Research Foundation, 2007). Based on recent surveys, employers do agree on the following issues:
· the need to take early action
· the need to clarify a diagnosis of "stress"
· a preference to keep employees working to prevent estrangement
· some willingness to be flexible with return-to-work arrangements
· the need to place limits on the amount of time off allowed.

Documenting prognosis

The key questions are: *"When is return to work expected?"* and *"What is the individual's prognosis for returning to work in his or her previous or modified position?"*

There are several prognostic indicators for a return to work after mental health disability. In determining prognosis, the clinician must consider a host of factors including clinical, psychosocial and workplace factors. Below are some of the most important factors (Dorian & Bender, 2010).

Clinical
· Premorbid functioning
· Severity of symptoms
· Motivation
· Duration of disability

Workplace
· Employer support
· Relationship and duration with employer
· Prior job satisfaction

Psychosocial
· Financial needs
· Pending litigation
· Support at home

When considering the factors related to documenting prognosis,
the key points for the primary care provider are:
· Prognosis for return to work decreases with time.
· Disability may be avoided if alternative work is available.
· Non-clinical factors are usually more important than clinical factors.

Conclusion
Mental health disability is a growing and challenging part of any medical
practice. Timely completion of forms and active management of disability
are the most important tasks for primary care providers. Coupled with
knowledge of the workplace and a focus on perceived barriers, prolonged
disability can often be avoided.

References

American Psychiatric Association. (2000). *Diagnostic and Statistical Manual of Mental Disorders* (4th ed., text rev.). Washington DC: Author.

Canadian Psychiatric Research Foundation. (2007). *When Something's Wrong: Strategies for Employers*. Toronto: Author.

Demeter, S.L. & Andersson, G.B.J. (2003). *Disability Evaluation* (2nd ed.). St. Louis, MO: Mosby.

Dorian, B.J. & Bender, A. (2010). Assessment of patients for insurance and disability. In D.S. Goldbloom (Ed.), *Psychiatric Clinical Skills* (Rev. 1st ed.; pp. 277–292). Toronto: Centre for Addiction and Mental Health.

Franche, R.L. & Krause, N. (2002). Readiness for return to work following injury or illness: Conceptualizing the interpersonal impact of health care, workplace, and insurance factors. *Journal of Occupational Rehabilitation, 12* (4), 233–256. DOI: 10.1023/A:1020270407044

Murray, C.J. & Lopez, A.D. (1997). Global mortality, disability, and the contribution of risk factors: Global Burden of Disease Study. *Lancet, 349* (9063), 1436–1442. DOI: 10.1016/S0140-6736(96)07495-8

Ontario Medical Association. (2007). *Physician's Guide to Third Party and Other Uninsured Services*. Toronto: Author.

World Health Organization (WHO). (1980). *International Classification of Impairments, Disabilities, and Handicaps*. Geneva, Switzerland: Author.

World Health Organization (WHO). (2001). *International Classification of Functioning, Disability and Health*. Geneva, Switzerland: Author.

16

Child and adolescent psychiatry

ALEXA BAGNELL

Introduction

Mental health concerns are a common reason for visiting a primary care setting. However, the diagnosis of these disorders in children and adolescents can be complicated and mental health treatments are often not readily accessible. To add to these difficulties, some of the medications used to treat common mental health problems in this age group have recently reported warnings related to serious side-effects. This can leave primary care clinicians feeling anxious and unsure about what to do to help the youth in their office presenting with mental health concerns. The goal of this chapter is to provide some guidelines and treatment recommendations for working with children and adolescents with mental health problems.

Setting the context

Confidentiality

It is important that the youth and the youth's family understand the limits of confidentiality. Confidentiality of information will be respected when possible, but if there is a risk of harm to self or others or significant safety concern, then confidentiality cannot be maintained. By saying this at the beginning, it prevents confusion and frustration, as well as loss of trust on the part of the child or adolescent, or the family.

An example of a confidentiality statement is: "What we talk about is confidential, which means I will keep what you say private and not share it with your parents or anyone else unless you are in agreement. However, if I have concerns about your safety or others' safety from what you tell me, I cannot keep that information private."

Every clinician has a different threshold for confidentiality. Although some situations for breaking confidentiality are clear (e.g., a youth confides that he or she is planning to take pills to end his or her life), some situations are less straightforward. If you are concerned about safety and will be informing parents/guardians, let the youth know beforehand, as this will help preserve the treatment relationship.

Family functioning
· What are the issues at home?
· How is the presenting problem affecting other family members?
· What is the level of family distress?
· What are the current supports?

School/academic functioning
· Are there any previous learning difficulties?
· What is academic functioning at present? Is this different than last year?
· Any school stressors?
· How is homework time?

Peers and social functioning
· How do they get along with peers?
· Have there been any changes in social group?
· What do they do outside of school?
· Any alcohol or other drug use, including smoking?

Child and adolescent psychiatry disorders

Attention-deficit/hyperactivity disorder
See also "The adult patient with ADHD" on page 191.

DIAGNOSTIC CLUES
Taking into account the developmental stage of the child, note if the child:
· has difficulty sitting still in your office and is climbing up on furniture
· constantly interrupts you or parents during conversation and has difficulty waiting for his or her turn to speak
· is not able to amuse himself or herself with toys in the office, constantly switching activities and asking questions
· draws attention to noises outside of office (e.g., frequently goes to the window or stops talking when there is a slight sound outside the office door).

KEY QUESTIONS
For parents
· Does your child have difficulty focusing on and completing tasks (video games, computer and television do not count)?
· Does your child lose things often or is your child forgetful (e.g., you have to repeat the same single instruction multiple times before he or she remembers to do it)?
· Is your child "always on the go" and does this interfere with things at home or school (e.g., sent to the principal's office for leaving his or her seat in the classroom repeatedly)?
· Is homework time a very difficult time in your house? How often does it not get completed because it is too stressful?
· Is your child having any difficulties socially due to interrupting others or not being able to wait for his or her turn?
· Were some of these difficulties present before your child was seven years old?

SCREENING TOOL
· The SNAP-IV Teacher and Parent Rating Scale (available online at http://adhd.net and through CADDRA's *Canadian ADHD Practice Guidelines*)

TREATMENT OPTIONS
· Psychostimulants (see page 293), non-stimulant medication (atomoxetine)
· Parent training in behaviour management strategies for ADHD
· School supports/classroom adaptations

MONITORING
· Medication evaluation (see page 292)
· Height, weight, blood pressure, heart rate. Patients should be comprehensively assessed if cardiac symptoms or risk factors are identified when prescribing ADHD medications.

RULE OUT
· Learning disorders, depressive disorders, anxiety disorders, disruptive behaviour disorders, and visual and auditory problems. Significant family dysfunction can present with symptoms of ADHD.

Depression
See also "The patient who is depressed" on page 13.

DIAGNOSTIC CLUES
When diagnosing depressive disorders in children and adolescents, the same criteria apply as for adults. The only differences in DSM-IV-TR criteria for children and adolescents is that mood may be irritable rather than depressed and that the duration of dysthymia is one year instead of two years as in adults. The primary care provider should also note:
· sad, restricted affect in office; may be tearful and/or irritable
· negative outlook and inability to identify anything that he or she enjoys or feels good about
· thinking of death and not wanting to live or "be around anymore," that "no one would notice," or everyone would be "better off" if he or she wasn't alive
· not future-oriented, no plans and no goals.

KEY QUESTIONS

For parents

- Does the child or adolescent cry excessively or complain of feeling sad most of the time?
- Has there been a noticeable change in school performance such as a drop in grades, poor work quality or not wanting to go to school?
- Has the child or adolescent stopped doing anything he or she used to enjoy?
- Is the child or adolescent more negative about himself/herself and others than before?
- Is the child or adolescent more easily angered and irritated by things that used not to bother him or her?
- Has there been any change in appetite, weight or sleep patterns?
- Does the child or adolescent have recurrent thoughts of suicide?

TREATMENT OPTIONS

- Selective serotonin reuptake inhibitors (SSRIs)
- Cognitive-behavioural therapy (CBT), interpersonal therapy (IPT)

MONITORING

- Physical exam and review of systems
- Thyroid screen and complete blood count (screen for anemia), other blood work as indicated by the physical exam and history
- Suicide risk and mania screen

RULE OUT

- Grief/bereavement, adjustment disorder (e.g., recent break-up of romantic relationship), substance use disorder and anxiety disorder. Significant family dysfunction can present with symptoms of depression.

Mania

See also "The patient who is manic" on page 27.

DIAGNOSTIC CLUES
- Pressured speech and difficult to interrupt during conversation
- Racing ideas, difficulty keeping track of topic or question asked
- Talking about abilities and capabilities as much greater than reality
- Easily distracted and agitated in office
- Affect that is very bright, euphoric and not consistent with the situation or material being discussed

KEY QUESTIONS
For the patient
- Have you had any period of several days or longer when you needed less sleep but still felt rested and energized?
- Have you found your thoughts are racing and difficult to keep track of?
- Do you have any special powers or abilities?
- Can you see or hear things that other people can't?
- Do your friends tell you that you are more talkative than usual and hard to have a conversation with or that you are difficult to understand?
- Have you done anything that is out of the ordinary for you and had the potential to cause serious problems for you?
- Have you had anger or aggression that is out of character for you?

SCREENING TOOL
- Young Mania Rating Scale (YMRS)

TREATMENT OPTIONS
- Mood stabilizers, atypical antipsychotics, benzodiazepines
- Cognitive-behavioural therapy (CBT)
- Family/patient education
- Referral to a specialist

MONITORING
- Physical exam and review of systems, screening blood work and toxicology screen, possibly brain imaging, ECG

RULE OUT
· Substance use disorder, adjustment disorder, disruptive behaviour disorder and ADHD. All can present with some symptoms of mania.

Anxiety
See also "The patient who is anxious" on page 45.

DIAGNOSTIC CLUES
Anxiety disorders in children and adolescents meet the same diagnostic criteria as adults with a few exceptions: children may lack insight into excessive or unreasonable nature of an anxiety reaction, and distress in children and adolescents may manifest behaviourally (i.e., crying, tantrum, freezing, agitation, clinging, refusal). Separation anxiety disorder and selective mutism are child-specific anxiety disorders. The primary care provider should also note:
· difficulty separating from parents during appointment
· trouble making eye contact and answering questions
· asking repetitive questions about same topic, seeking reassurance
· shaking legs, trembling hands, fidgeting or crying.

KEY QUESTIONS
For the patient
Younger children usually relate to the term "worry" better than "anxiety."
· Do you worry more than other kids you know?
· Does worry/fear/anxiety ever stop you from doing something that you would like to be able to do?
· Do you sleep in your own bed all night?
· What do you worry about?
· Have you ever missed school or had to come home from school early?
· Have you ever had anxiety where your heart raced, you couldn't catch your breath, you felt dizzy or lightheaded and thought you might be dying?
· Do you get a lot of stomach aches and headaches?
· Describe your sleep routine.
· Do you have trouble concentrating?

· Do you have any routines or behaviours you need to do to relieve anxiety or upsetting thoughts or images? (For example, ask about germs/dirt worries and handwashing/cleaning, also counting and checking rituals.)
· What would be different for you if you didn't have anxiety/worry?

SCREENING TOOLS
· Screen for Child Anxiety Related Emotional Disorders (SCARED)

TREATMENT OPTIONS
· Cognitive-behavioural therapy (CBT)
· Selective serotonin reuptake inhibitors (SSRIs)

MONITORING
· Physical exam and review of systems, medical work-up as indicated

RULE OUT
· Depressive disorder, ADHD, family or social stressor, and learning disorder. All can present with some symptoms of anxiety.

Psychosis
See also "The patient who is psychotic" on page 113.

DIAGNOSTIC CLUES
· Distracted and staring off in office, requiring questions repeated
· Difficulty following conversation, jumping topics, not making sense
· Agitation and irritability, distrust, guarded, suspicious
· Blunted affect, dishevelled, poor hygiene
· Paucity of speech
· Repetitive or rigid thinking
· Reports no problems when there is evidence of significant impairment (lack of insight)
· Prodromal warning signs (social withdrawal, intense preoccupations, day/night sleep reversal)

Youth with psychotic-like episodes (PLE) (psychotic symptoms episodic and/or transient, such as once per month, and other symptoms of psychosis not present) and youth with prodromal symptoms (social withdrawal, unusual behaviour, decline in personal hygiene, difficulty concentrating) may be at higher risk of developing a psychotic illness and periodic monitoring of symptoms is recommended.

KEY QUESTIONS
For the patient
- Do you ever see, hear, smell or feel things that other people do not?
- Do you ever feel like your thoughts are being controlled by someone or something else?
- Do you ever feel that someone wishes to harm you or is out to get you?
- Do you have any special powers or abilities (e.g., can you control others' thoughts, are there special messages for you through the television, can you communicate with God)?

For parents
- Have there been any unusual or unexplained changes in behaviour?
- Are there any problems at school or with friends?

SCREENING TOOL
- Positive and Negative Syndrome Scale (PANSS)

TREATMENT OPTIONS
- Youth and family education and support
- Antipsychotic medication (atypical and typical antipsychotics)
- Cognitive-behavioural therapy (CBT)
- Minimization of relapse risk (e.g., treatment of substance abuse, anxiety, mood disorder)
- Referral to a specialist

INVESTIGATION
- First episode: full medical work-up including brain imaging

MONITORING SIDE-EFFECTS OF ANTIPSYCHOTICS
· Height, weight, blood pressure, waist circumference
· Lab: fasting lipids, fasting blood glucose and prolactin on atypical antipsychotic
· ECG as indicated

Eating disorder

See also "The patient with an eating disorder" on page 129.

DIAGNOSTIC CLUES
· Thin or emaciated facial appearance
· Wearing warmer clothes than indicated by season
· Reports worries about being fat when not overweight
· Loss of significant amount of weight in relatively short time
· Loss of menstrual cycle

KEY QUESTIONS
For the patient
· Does your weight affect how you feel about yourself? How often do you weigh yourself?
· Are you satisfied with your eating patterns? Do you diet?
· Do you ever make yourself sick when you feel uncomfortably full?
· Do you believe that you are fat when others say you are thin?
· Have you lost any weight in the last three months? Do you think you need to lose weight? How much?
· Do you ever skip meals? What did you have for lunch?
· What is your current exercise routine?

For parents
· Does your child go to the bathroom immediately after eating?
· Does your child have any unusual eating behaviours (e.g., hiding food, cutting food into very small pieces, moving food around on the plate but not eating it)?

SCREENING TOOL
· SCOFF Eating Disorders Questionnaire (Morgan et al., 1999)

TREATMENT OPTIONS
· Youth and family education and therapy
· Meal support (family training in supervising meals)
· Limit exercise, bathroom access after meals
· Referral to a specialist

MONITORING
· Physical exam, height, weight, blood pressure and heart rate (lying/sitting)
· Blood work: complete blood count with differential, thyroid screen, electrolytes (K, Na, Cl, HCO_3), liver enzymes, Ca, Mg
· ECG

Psychopharmacology

This section provides prescribing and monitoring guidelines for stimulant, antidepressant and atyptical antipsychotic medications.

Psychostimulants

INDICATIONS
· Attention-deficit/hyperactivity disorder (ADHD)

WARNINGS
· There is increased risk of cardiac event and possible sudden death in children and adolescents with cardiac risk factors (structural cardiac abnormality, cardiac disease, hyperthyroidism, heart conduction problems, family history of sudden cardiac death).

RECOMMENDED MONITORING
· Review history, physical exam and family history to assess cardiac risk.
· Monitor height, weight, blood pressure and heart rate at baseline and follow-up visits.

· Assess patients comprehensively if cardiac symptoms or risk factors are identified when prescribing ADHD medications. In Canada there is an advisory warning (Health Canada, 2006) regarding use of stimulant and non-stimulant (atomoxetine) medication in youth with cardiac symptoms or disease, hyperthyroidism, structural cardiac abnormalities, or family history of sudden cardiac death. Cardiology work-up as indicated is first recommended in these cases.

MOST COMMON SIDE-EFFECTS

· Decreased appetite, insomnia, irritability, anxiety and sadness are common side-effects.
· Hyperactive rebound can occur in afternoon or evening particularly with short-acting stimulants and may be helped by changing dosage timing or switching to slow-release preparation.

ABUSE RISK

· Stimulant medications all carry risk of abuse if misused. However, children with treated ADHD are significantly less likely to abuse substances than those with untreated ADHD.
· Shorter acting/immediate release forms have slightly higher risk of abuse. Not advised for those with history of substance abuse. Consider the non-stimulant medication atomoxetine.

Antidepressants

INDICATIONS

· Fluoxetine is the only SSRI approved (U.S., U.K.) for treatment of depression (ages 8–17 years).
· Fluoxetine, sertraline and fluvoxamine are approved (U.S.) for OCD (ages 8–17 years).
· Atomoxetine is approved (U.S. and Canada) for ADHD.

WARNINGS

· In 2004, a Health Canada warning and FDA box warning was issued for all antidepressants in youth 18 years of age and under: Risk of increased

suicidal ideation and behaviour (not suicide) with antidepressant medication. However, depression and other serious mental illnesses are the most important causes of suicide. Current research supports antidepressant treatment of moderate to severe depression and/or anxiety in this age group, as the benefit of treatment of these serious mental illnesses outweighs the risk of suicidal ideation/behaviour associated with the antidepressants (Bridge et al., 2007).
· Consensus is to treat the illness if risks of untreated illness are clinically significant and monitor closely for medication side-effects. The current recommendation is treatment of moderate to severe depression with an antidepressant (first choice: fluoxetine). Risk of suicidal behaviours is thought to be highest in the first several months of treatment and after any increases in dosage.

RECOMMENDED MONITORING
· Prior to initiating antidepressant medication, inform all patients and families of potential side-effects and the Health Canada warning regarding increased risk of suicidal ideation and behaviour.
· Follow up with appointments every one to two weeks with starting medication or after an increase in dosage. Inform families to call if they have concerns regarding medication.
· Start at the lowest dose range and increase slowly. Many children and adolescents respond to a lower dosage range of antidepressants.
· Antidepressants take several weeks to start working and have continued improvement for about 12 weeks at that dosage.
· Recommend continuing the antidepressant for six to 12 months after symptoms resolve before discontinuing.
· Inform patients of discontinuation syndrome: withdrawal side-effects (increased agitation, irritability, flu-like symptoms, paresthesias, dizziness) if medication is stopped abruptly. These occur most commonly in antidepressants with a short half-life such as paroxetine and venlafaxine and can be reduced by gradually tapering off the medication.
· Some antidepressants are associated with weight gain (e.g., paroxetine), and monitoring height and weight is suggested.

MOST COMMON SIDE-EFFECTS
· GI distress (recommend taking with food), insomnia, drowsiness/sedation, headache, dry mouth, dizziness, sexual disturbances, excitement/hypomania, fatigue and tremor are common side-effects.

Atypical antipsychotics

INDICATIONS
· No approved indications in children and adolescents. Therefore the clinical use is off-label and their use should be justified with a clinical note.
· In adults indications include psychosis, schizophrenia, bipolar disorder, mania, agitation/aggression.

WARNINGS
· Weight gain. Aripiprazole and ziprasidone are associated with the least weight gain. Olanzapine is associated with the most weight gain.
· Hyperprolactinemia: amenorrhea, gynecomastia, galactorrhea (risperidone has the highest risk).
· Metabolic syndrome includes obesity, disturbed glucose or insulin metabolism, lipid dysregulation, hypertension (aripiprazole has the lowest risk).
· Extrapyramidal side-effects (dystonia, dyskinesia, akathisia) are less common in atypical antipsychotics and are dose dependent (increased risk at higher medication dosages and in youth with developmental disabilities). The use of risperidone is associated with the highest rates of extrapyramidal side-effects.
· ECG changes (e.g., prolongation of QTc interval) may increase risk of arrhythmia.
· Lower seizure threshold. Caution in patients with history of seizures.
· Tardive dyskinesia. Risk is much lower with atypical antipsychotics.
· Dystonic reactions are less frequent in atypical antipsychotics (less than 2 per cent). Note: Acute dystonia with difficulty swallowing or trouble breathing is a medical emergency.

RECOMMENDED MONITORING
- Inform all patients and families of potential side-effects.
- Monitor height, weight, waist circumference, heart rate and blood pressure at baseline and follow-up appointments.
- Monitor blood work at baseline and every four to six months: lipid profile, blood glucose, prolactin, ECG.
- Taper medication over weeks or months after prolonged use. Stopping medication abruptly, or a significant decrease in dosage, can cause discontinuation syndrome within a few days and withdrawal dyskinesia (common in children) within one to four weeks.
- Most common side-effects include weight gain, sedation, dizziness, fatigue, headache, insomnia/agitation, dysphoria, orthostatic hypotension, sexual dysfunction, anticholinergic side-effects.

Crisis management

Managing suicidal thoughts and behaviour
If a child or adolescent discloses or endorses thoughts of ending his or her life or not wanting to live, there must be an assessment of suicide risk.

SUICIDE RISK ASSESSMENT
Suicide risk factors
- Mental illness (e.g., major depressive disorder)
- Substance abuse
- Prior suicide attempt
- Family history of suicide and suicide attempts
- Involvement of juvenile justice system

Ways to ask about suicidal thoughts, behaviours and intent
- Have you ever felt life was not worth living?
- Have you ever tried to do something to harm yourself that could have seriously harmed you or killed you?
- Do you currently have a plan to kill yourself?
- Would you act on this plan? Why or why not?
- What would happen if you followed through on this plan?

Assessing environment

· What are the current stressors in your life?
· Who do you talk to?
· What would you do if you needed help?

Suicidal intent or a failed attempt

The intent to attempt suicide or a failed suicide attempt is a psychiatric emergency. The patient should, if possible, be assessed in an emergency room as observation and/or admission for safety may be required.

Managing acute psychosis

It is a medical emergency if a child or youth presents with a sudden onset of psychotic symptoms such as hallucinations, delusions, bizarre and disorganized behaviour, incomprehensible speech or extreme paranoia.

SAFETY

First address the question, is this youth a safety risk to self or others in his or her current mental state? If there is extreme agitation or aggression, then medication may be required. First, check if there is any information regarding drug intoxication or reaction that may be the cause of current symptoms as this may guide what medication to use.

Benzodiazepines (e.g., lorazepam 0.5–2 mg sl or po) are often given to help calm patients in this situation. Occasionally, when oral medication cannot be administered due to extreme agitation and refusal, i.m. medication is used, including benzodiazepines (e.g., lorazepam 0.5–2 mg i.m.) and antipsychotics (e.g., haloperidol 1–5 mg i.m., olanzapine 2.5–5 mg i.m.).

The youth should be transported to an emergency room for medical work-up as soon as possible.

Managing aggression/agitation

Aggression or agitation is a sign that a child or adolescent is having difficulty coping with something in the immediate environment. Take a break from the topic being discussed and assess the situation. Make sure the environment (e.g., office) is a safe place to continue or move to another area.

Ask the youth what would be helpful in the present situation. Remove stressors if possible (e.g., request that parent or sibling leave the room).

If aggression and agitation escalate and the situation becomes a safety concern, the youth may need medication (e.g., lorazepam 0.5 – 2 mg sl or po).

For extremely agitated and dangerous behaviour, see "Managing acute psychosis" above.

Special topics in child and adolescent mental health

Sleep
See also "The patient with a sleep disorder" on page 207.

Sleep is a common concern of parents, children and youth. Preschool children should sleep about 12 to 14 hours per night. School-age children should sleep about 10 to 12 hours per night. Adolescents should sleep about 9 hours per night.

Some mental health problems (e.g., anxiety, depression) have related sleep problems. With treatment of the disorder, sleep improves, and improvement in sleep can lead to improved mental health.

SLEEP HYGIENE TECHNIQUES
- Regular bedtime and wake time (weeknights and weekdays)
- No screens (TV, computer, games) in room, or turn off at least one hour before bedtime; no lights on in room
- Regular exercise at least four to five times per week (at least two hours before bedtime)
- Relaxing music, relaxation exercises, or reading as pre-bedtime routine

· No daytime naps
· No caffeinated beverages after 1:00 p.m.
· No big meals or spicy or high-sugar foods before bedtime

SLEEP MEDICATION
Medication for sleep should only be used if sleep hygiene techniques are not working or sleep issues are a significant factor in a mental health disorder. Medication should be used only for a short amount of time to get the sleep cycle back on track and then efforts should be made to discontinue.

Diphenhydramine
· 12.5 to 50 mg qhs
· Can have paradoxical reaction in children with increased hyperactivity and agitation
· Most common side-effects: sedation, fatigue, incoordination, insomnia, GI disturbance, dry mouth, blurred vision, confusion, delirium

Zopiclone
· 3.75 to 15 mg qhs
· Safety and efficacy not established in pediatric age group
· Low risk of dependence
· Most common side-effects: bitter metallic taste, dry mouth, GI distress, severe drowsiness, confusion, palpitations, tremor, chills/sweats, agitation, incoordination, dyspnea, nightmares

Melatonin
· 1.5 to 3 mg "natural supplement"
· Evidence mixed as to effectiveness
· Short-term use of up to several weeks has safety data
· Not recommended in patients with autoimmune disorders
· Most common side-effects: fatigue, dizziness, headache, increased irritability, abdominal cramps at high dosages

Trazodone
- 25 to 50 mg qhs
- No approved indications in children and adolescents; therefore, the clinical use is off-label and should be justified with a clinical note.
- Can cause priapism in males, which is a medical emergency
- ECG changes and cardiac arrhythmia: use with caution if pre-existing cardiac disease
- Most common side-effects: drowsiness, fatigue, dry mouth, dizziness/ orthostatic hypotension, GI distress, headache, weight gain, blurred vision, constipation, tremor, insomnia

Bullying
Bullying is common in youth and has a significant negative impact on mental health. Bullying includes physical (e.g., hitting, punching), verbal (e.g., name calling), indirect (e.g., exclusion) and cyber (Internet, instant messaging) bullying. Parents should be encouraged to take bullying seriously, listen and empathize with their child, and work with the school and community to address bullying issues. Parents should also encourage children to protect their personal information and understand what appropriate communication on the Internet is.

Children and youth should be encouraged to tell a trusted adult if they are being bullied and to report the bullying of others. Emphasis should be on supporting the youth being bullied and working toward a solution within the environment, with recognition that sometimes this can take some time.

Young people who are being bullied should be encouraged to stay close to friends, walk away from difficult situations if possible, and avoid places where they are more likely to be targeted.

Learning disorders
Learning disorders can present with mental health symptoms such as depression and anxiety. Children and youth with learning disorders have

higher rates of mental health problems (e.g., 20 to 30 per cent of youth with ADHD have a comorbid learning disorder).

Learning disorders should be considered if the symptoms are specific to the school situation, or if a child or adolescent is struggling academically and not progressing as expected in school. To be diagnosed, learning disorders require testing. This testing can be accessed by referring the child or youth to a psychologist—either through the school system (parents can also request this from school) or in the community—who has the training to administer and evaluate these tests.

Pervasive developmental disorders

Autism and autism spectrum disorders (Asperger's disorder, pervasive developmental disorder) require a full diagnostic test administered by a trained specialist to be accurately diagnosed. Refer to a specialist if there is a significant concern regarding a child's communication skills, social interaction or behaviours consistent with a pervasive developmental disorder.

Addictions

See also "The patient who is abusing substances" on page 85.

Problems with substance use and misuse commonly begin in adolescence. All youth should be asked about alcohol and other drug use (including the use of tobacco), how much and how often, and whether it has caused them any problems in their life.

There is high comorbidity between substance use disorders and mental health disorders. Substance abuse is a risk factor for suicide. Treatment of concurrent mental health and substance use disorders usually requires referral to specialty mental health services that address both addiction and mental health treatment.

Most substance use disorders, including dependence, can be effectively treated in primary care.

When to refer to a specialist

· Severe symptom presentation:
  - acute psychosis
  - mania
  - depression with serious suicidality
  - severe eating disorder
  - severe obsessive-compulsive disorder
· Significant comorbidity:
  - substance abuse, aggressive disruptive and dangerous behaviour, autism, psychosis
· Diagnostic clarification:
  - psychosis
  - bipolar disorder in youth
  - learning disorder
  - pervasive developmental disorders
· Treatment resistance
  - if two trials of medication have failed or if recommended psychotherapy has failed

Community and online resources

Mental health supports

· Hospital and university psychiatry outpatient and inpatient services
· Community health/mental health clinic: psychologists, social workers, psychiatrists, pediatricians
· Department of Community Services or child welfare service

Resources for primary practitioners

· National Institute of Mental Health. Information on child and adolescent mental illnesses and treatment: www.nimh.nih.gov/health/topics/child-and-adolescent-mental-health/index.shtml
· Canadian Mental Health Association. Information on resources available across Canada: www.cmha.ca

Resources for families

- Canadian Psychiatric Research Foundation: *When Something's Wrong: Ideas for Families* and *When Something's Wrong: Strategies for Teachers*. The handbooks cover common mental health problems in children and adolescents. Downloadable from www.cprf.ca
- American Academy of Child and Adolescent Psychiatry: Facts for Families. The site contains a range of information on mental health issues, along with information on topics as diverse as bedwetting, violence on television and sex education. Downloadable from www.aacap.org
- Canadian Psychological Association: "Psychology Works" fact sheets cover a broad range of mental health issues, including information related to children and adolescents. Downloadable from www.cpa.ca/psychologyfactsheets/
- Schoolpsychiatry.org (Massachusetts General Hospital): Resources for parents, educators and clinicians with a special emphasis on supporting youth with mental health disorders in school. Downloadable from http://www.massgeneral.org/schoolpsychiatry/
- National Alliance on Mental Illness: NAMI offers information for patients and families on a range of mental health problems. Downloadable from www.nami.org

References

American Psychiatric Association. (2000). *Diagnostic and Statistical Manual of Mental Disorders* (4th ed., text rev.). Washington DC: Author.

Barrett, P.M. & Ollendick, T.H. (Eds.). (2004). *Handbook of Interventions that Work with Children and Adolescents: Prevention and Treatment*. West Sussex, England: John Wiley & Sons.

Bezchlibnyk-Butler K.Z. & Virani, A.S. (2007). *Clinical Handbook of Psychotropic Drugs for Children and Adolescents* (2nd revised and expanded edition). Cambridge, MA: Hogrefe & Huber.

Bridge, J.A., Iyengar, S., Salary, C.B., Barbe, R.P., Birmaher, B., Pincus, H.A. et al. (2007). Clinical response and risk for reported suicidal ideation and suicide attempts in pediatric antidepressant treatment: A meta-analysis of randomized controlled trials. *Journal of the American Medical Association, 297* (15), 1683–1696. DOI: 10.1001/jama.297.15.1683

Health Canada. (2006). *Attention Deficit Hyperactivity Disorder (ADHD) Drugs: Updated and Standardized Labelling Regarding Very Rare Cardiac-Related Adverse Events* [Health Products and Food Branch Advisory, May 2006]. Retrieved from http://www.hc-sc.gc.ca/dhp-mps/medeff/advisories-avis/prof/_2006/adhd-tdah_medic_hpc-cps-eng.php

Hill, L.S., Reid, F., Morgan, J.F. & Lacey, J.H. (2010). SCOFF, the development of an eating disorder screening questionnaire. *International Journal of Eating Disorders, 43* (4), 344 –351. DOI:10.1002/eat.20679

Martin, A., Volkmar, F.R. & Lewis, M. (2007). *Lewis' Child and Adolescent Psychiatry. A Comprehensive Textbook* (4th ed.). Philadelphia, PA: Lippincott, Williams and Wilkins.

Morgan, J.F., Reid, F. & Lacey, J.H. (1999). The SCOFF questionnaire: Assessment of a new screening tool for eating disorders. *British Medical Journal, 319,* 1467–1468.

National Institute of Mental Health. (n.d.). Health and Outreach: Child and Adolescent Mental Health [Website information]. Retrieved from http://www.nimh.nih.gov/health/topics/child-and-adolescent-mental-health/index.shtml

Vetter, V.L., Elia, J., Erickson, C., Berger, S., Blum, N., Uzark, K. et al. (2008). Cardiovascular monitoring of children and adolescents with heart disease receiving stimulant drugs: A scientific statement from the American Heart Association Congenital Cardiac Defects Committee of the Council on Cardiovascular Disease in the Young and the Council on Cardiovascular Nursing. *Circulation, 117,* 2407–2423. DOI: 10.1161/CIRCULATIONAHA.107.189473

17

Perinatal mood and anxiety disorders

SHAILA MISRI AND ANNA LEHMAN

Overview

Mood disorders in the perinatal period

EPIDEMIOLOGY
- 10 to 15 per cent of women will experience depression in the perinatal period.
- Nearly half of women with a prior history of depression will relapse in the perinatal period.
- More than half of patients diagnosed with depression in the postpartum period have the onset of illness in pregnancy.
- Three per cent of pregnant women use SSRIs.

CLINICAL PRESENTATION
- Pregnancy does not offer protection from mental illness.
- Signs of pregnancy and depression overlap.
- Depression can present with either agitation or retardation.

Anxiety disorders in the perinatal period

EPIDEMIOLOGY
- Over half of women with depression have a concurrent anxiety disorder.

CLINICAL PRESENTATION
- Anxiety disorders may present as panic disorder, generalized anxiety disorder, obsessive-compulsive disorder, phobias, and posttraumatic stress disorder.
- Acute symptoms drive women to seek medical attention.

Risk factors for mood and anxiety disorders

Biological
- Past history of depression
- Past history of postpartum depression—up to 50 per cent recurrence for subsequent pregnancies
- Family history of mental illness—first-degree relative doubles the risk
- Recent discontinuation of antidepressants—75 per cent relapse
- Medical or obstetrical problems
- Substance abuse

Psychosocial
- An unplanned pregnancy or ambivalent feelings about the pregnancy
- Marital discord
- Personality traits—for example, perfectionism
- Return-to-work pressures
- Sexual, physical, emotional abuse
- Lower socioeconomic status, financial difficulties
- Recent immigration

Consequences of untreated perinatal mood and anxiety disorders

Maternal consequences
- Progression of the mental illness
- Poor prenatal care

- Risk of medical/obstetrical complications such as gestational diabetes, premature labour
- Self-medication/substance abuse
- Impaired bonding/maternal-infant interaction
- Suicide/infanticide

Neonatal consequences
- Preterm delivery
- Poor neonatal adaptation—altered sleep, increased irritability, crying, lethargy
- Lower birth weight (associated with increased uterine artery resistance)
- Greater right frontal EEG activation
- Lower dopamine and serotonin levels
- Lower scores on Brazelton Neonatal Behavioral Assessment Scale

Childhood and adolescent consequences
- Anxiety/depression, withdrawal, somatic complaints (internalizing behaviours)
- ADHD, aggression in boys, rule-breaking (externalizing behaviours)
- Increased impulsivity
- Lower scores on WISC-R intelligence subtests

Assessment of "postpartum blues"
- Experienced by 50 to 85 per cent of women
- Transient, mild symptoms
- No loss of functionality
- Self-limited to two weeks
- No major intervention required

Assessment of depressive disorders

Screening
· Edinburgh Postnatal Depression Scale — a validated self-rated tool
  (see below)
· Screening at 28–32 weeks of gestation and again six to eight weeks postpartum
· Frequent screening for high-risk population

Edinburgh Postnatal Depression Scale

As you have recently had a baby, we would like to know how you are feeling. Please
UNDERLINE the answer which comes closest to how you have felt IN THE PAST
7 DAYS, not just how you feel today.

1. I have been able to laugh and see the funny side of things.
    As much as I always could
    Not quite so much now
    Definitely not so much now
    Not at all

2. I have looked forward with enjoyment to things.
    As much as I ever did
    Rather less than I used to
    Definitely less than I used to
    Hardly at all

*3. I have blamed myself unnecessarily when things went wrong.
    Yes, most of the time
    Yes, some of the time
    Not very often
    No, never

4. I have been anxious or worried for no good reason.
    No, not at all
    Hardly ever
    Yes, sometimes
    Yes, very often

*5. I have felt scared or panicky for not very good reason.
    Yes, quite a lot
    Yes, sometimes
    No, not much
    No, not at all

*6. Things have been getting on top of me.
    Yes, most of the time I haven't been able to cope at all
    Yes, sometimes I haven't been coping as well as usual
    No, most of the time I have coped quite well
    No, I have been coping as well as ever

*7. I have been so unhappy that I have had difficulty sleeping.
    Yes, most of the time
    Yes, sometimes
    Not very often
    No, not at all

*8. I have felt sad or miserable.
    Yes, most of the time
    Yes, quite often
    Not very often
    No, not at all

*9. I have been so unhappy that I have been crying.
    Yes, most of the time
    Yes, quite often
    Only occasionally
    No, never

*10. The thought of harming myself has occurred to me.
    Yes, quite often
    Sometimes
    Hardly ever
    Never

Response categories are scored 0, 1, 2, and 3 according to increased severity of the symptoms. Items marked with an asterisk are reverse scored (i.e. 3, 2, 1, and 0). The total score is calculated by adding together the scores for each of the 10 items. A score > 13 indicates depression likely.

Reproduced with permission from: Cox, J.L., Holden, J.M. & Sagovsky, R. (1987). Detection of postnatal depression. Development of the 10-item Edinburgh Postnatal Depression Scale. *British Journal of Psychiatry, 150,* 782–786. Copyright 1987 The Royal College of Psychiatrists.

Clinician interview

· Review inventory of symptoms of depressive disorders as per DSM (see page 15).
· Take a personal psychiatric history, family psychiatric history.
· Assess premenstrual/contraceptive/seasonal-related mood changes.
· Assess suicidality (see "Assessment and management of suicide risk," page 237).
· Exclude medical morbidity (e.g., anemia, thyroid, renal, hepatic disease).
· Assess substance use (see "The patient with a substance use problem," page 85).
· Assess supports including partner, family and social supports.
· Ask about bonding (both during pregnancy and after).
· Observe maternal-infant interaction.

Assessment of postpartum psychosis

· Rare occurrence (1–2 /1000)
· Rapid development of delusions and hallucinations, labile mood and behaviour, and agitation in the first few weeks after delivery
· Psychiatric emergency that requires hospitalization
· Assess suicidal and homicidal potential
· Often the first presentation of bipolar disorder

Assessment of anxiety disorders

All pre-existing anxiety disorders may worsen in the perinatal period.

Panic disorder

· This is the most common presentation.

- Look for unusual/unrelated somatic complaints (see "The patient who is somatizing or is bodily preoccupied," page 61).
- Ask about ER/walk-in clinic visits.

Generalized anxiety disorder
- This is commonly missed.
- Look for excessive worry ("What if …?"), constantly seeking reassurance, catastrophizing events.

Obsessive-compulsive disorder
- This frightening condition often involves horrific intrusive thoughts of harming the baby or self.
- Reassure the patient since the risk of acting on these thoughts is extremely small.
- Look for worsening of pre-existing OCD.

Principles of management

Mild to moderate depression and anxiety
CONSIDER PSYCHOTHERAPY
Cognitive-behavioral therapy (CBT)
- CBT is best administered by CBT-trained providers.
- Monitor effectiveness/sustainability of treatment regularly.

Interpersonal therapy (IPT)
- Refer to an experienced counsellor.
- IPT is effective in women with problems with role-transition.

CONSIDER BIOMEDICAL INTERVENTION
Light therapy
- Light therapy is most effective for those with seasonal mood variation.
- Recommend trial with commercially available light boxes.

CONSIDER LIFESTYLE AND PERSONAL HEALTH INTERVENTIONS
· Increased support (i.e., help of partner, family and friends)
· Nutritious meals—address any disordered eating
· Sleep—suggest help with nighttime feedings
· Hydration
· Daily light exercise
· Focus on personal time

Moderate to severe depression and/or anxiety

CONSIDER PHARMACOTHERAPY
Ideally, pharmacotherapy should be accompanied by psychotherapy.

Discuss exposure of the fetus to medications versus mental illness
· No decision is risk-free.
· If conception occurs on antidepressant medication, a decision to discontinue
  must be weighed against a three to five times greater rate of relapse.
· Discuss in depth warnings regarding neonatal withdrawal (Moses-Kokol
  et al., 2005), paroxetine (GlaxoSmithKline, 2005), and persistent pulmonary
  hypertension of the newborn (PPHN) (Chambers et al., 2006), focusing on
  their merits versus methodological challenges:
  - Long-term studies up to six years of age show no cognitive effects of
    in utero exposure to SSRIs.
  - Exposure to persistent postpartum depression is associated with delayed
    language and cognitive development.
  - Treating maternal depression/anxiety helps prevent these outcomes
    in their children.
· Help the patient make an informed decision without bias.

Inform patients
The primary care provider should inform patients:
· of placental transfer of medication
· to continue nursing on the same medications used in pregnancy
· of excretion of medication into breast milk, which is generally negligible—
  a physician should monitor the breastfed infant.

Choice of pharmacotherapy
- No specific pharmacotherapy is "the best."
- Pharmacotherapy effective in the past is likely to work again.
- Recommend pharmacotherapy that has been effective for the patient's family members.
- Check for interactions with other medications.
- Perinatal patients often fail to respond to antidepressants alone.
- Augmentation with other medications, including antipsychotics, is useful for non-responders.
- Use benzodiazepines for no more than two weeks to stabilize extreme anxiety.
- Patients vary in response time/dose.

Compliance and discussion of side-effects
- Inform the patient that the most common side-effects — mild headache, GI upset — usually abate within one to two weeks.
- Advise the patient to avoid alcohol.
- Advise the patient that alternative therapies (e.g., St. John's wort) may adversely interact with medications.
- Advise against abrupt discontinuation. Slow taper is recommended.

Dose adjustment in pregnancy and postpartum
- Watch for mood changes in the late second and early third trimester.
- Dose increase may be required as plasma volume and hepatic metabolism change.

Duration of treatment
- For a single episode of depression, continue treatment for one year.
- Recurrent depressive episodes will likely require much longer-term maintenance therapy.

Psychosis and suicidality
Consider the following in acutely suicidal/psychotic pregnant and post-partum patients and explain the pros and cons to family members:
- emergency psychiatric consultation
- hospitalization
- ECT.

Table 17.1 Medications: Off-label Indications and Risks

PREGNANCY CATEGORY	DRUG AND DOSAGES: INITIAL AND MAXIMUM	INDICATIONS (OFF LABEL IN PREGNANCY)	COMMON MATERNAL ADVERSE EFFECTS (>4%)
SSRIs			
			Adverse effects are similar for all SSRIs. During the first few weeks, headache and nausea are common, but improve over time. Occasionally, insomnia, sexual dysfunction, weight gain and jitteriness may necessitate a switch.
C*	**Fluoxetine** 10–60 mg po q am Increase, if necessary, at intervals of ≥ 1 wk.	Depression Anxiety disorders	Rash, sweating, weight changes, GI disturbance, anxiety, sexual dysfunction
D**	**Paroxetine** 20–60 mg po q am Increase, if necessary, at intervals of ≥ 1 wk.	Depression Anxiety disorders	Sweating, GI disturbance, arthralgia, dizziness, insomnia, somnolence, tremor, blurred vision, agitation, impaired sexual functioning

FETAL EFFECTS	LACTATION
This class of medications may have an increased risk of respiratory distress, low birth weight and prematurity, proportionate to length of exposure. Neonatal withdrawal/toxicity (jitteriness, increased startle, jaundice, hypoglycemia, hypertonicity, feeding difficulties, and convulsions) is well documented (though usually mild) when exposure occurs late in pregnancy. Typically recovery ensues within 48 hours, and rarely lasts several weeks. There appear to be no long-term neurodevelopmental sequelae (unlike exposure to maternal depression). There may be association with heart defects, craniosynostosis, omphalocele, neural tube defects and anal atresia, although the absolute risk in studies remains small (i.e., odds ratios range 1.2 – 4 for generally rare anomalies).	There are no known serious side-effects for infants breastfeeding from mothers on an SSRI.
This agent has the most prospective data available for SSRIs in pregnancies. No confirmed increased risk of malformations. See above warnings on withdrawal symptoms and possible persistent pulmonary hypertension.	There is a small amount of the drug and its active metabolite excreted into breast milk (6.7%). There may be an association with reduced infant growth.
There is suggestive evidence of teratogenicity in first-trimester use of this medication and a Health Canada warning is in effect. Most commonly, the associated defect has been septal defects and, more rarely, right ventricular outflow track defects; fetal echocardiography may be appropriate if there is exposure in the first trimester. See above warnings regarding neonatal withdrawal and pulmonary hypertension of the newborn.	In infants of breastfeeding mothers taking paroxetine, serum drug levels are practically undetectable. The mean dose of exposure is estimated as 1.3% of the maternal weight-adjusted dose.

Table 17.1 Medications: Off-label, continued

PREGNANCY CATEGORY	DRUG AND DOSAGES: INITIAL AND MAXIMUM	INDICATIONS (OFF LABEL IN PREGNANCY)	COMMON MATERNAL ADVERSE EFFECTS (>4%)
C	**Sertraline** 25–200 mg/d po Increase, if necessary, at intervals of ≥ 1 wk.	Depression Anxiety disorders *Effective in RCT compared to placebo for postnatal depression.	Sweating, GI disturbance, dry mouth, myalgia, dizziness, headache, somnolence, agitation, sexual dysfunction
C	**Citalopram** 20–60 mg/d po Escitalopram 10–20 mg/d po Increase, if necessary, at intervals of ≥ 1 wk.	Depression Anxiety disorders	Dizziness, dry skin, somnolence, confusion
SNRIs			
C	**Venlafaxine** 75 mg/d po Max: 300 mg/d Increase, if necessary, at intervals of ≥ 1 wk.	Depression Anxiety disorders	Hypertension, sweating, weight change, GI disturbance, headache, dizziness, blurred vision, agitation, sleep disturbance
C	**Mirtazapine** 15mg/d po qhs Max: 45 mg/d Increase, if necessary, at intervals of ≥ 1 wk.	Depression	Hyperphagia, somnolence, elevated lipids, dizziness

FETAL EFFECTS	LACTATION
No confirmed increased malformation risk, although there is a reported association with omphalocele. Lower cord blood levels than citalopram or fluoxetine. See previous warnings on neonatal pulmonary hypertension and neonatal withdrawal.	Sertraline blood level in breastfeeding infants is nearly undetectable.
High risk of malformations is unlikely. There is no data specifically on escitalopram, but if the patient has already had an adequate response to it, then continue during the perinatal period. See previous warnings on neonatal pulmonary hypertension and neonatal withdrawal.	Infant serum levels are usually undetectable. The dose transmitted has been estimated at 4% of the maternal dose.
Little is known about risks, but no increased malformation risk has been established. Transient neonatal withdrawal after third trimester has been reported (jitteriness, hypertonia, poor feeding, irritability).	Breastfeeding infant serum levels are low.
One study shows increased rate of preterm delivery. There may also be an increased rate of spontaneous miscarriage. No increased malformation risk.	Very little is known.

Table 17.1 Medications: Off-label, continued

PREGNANCY CATEGORY	DRUG AND DOSAGES: INITIAL AND MAXIMUM	INDICATIONS (OFF LABEL IN PREGNANCY)	COMMON MATERNAL ADVERSE EFFECTS (>4%)
Atypical antidepressants			
C	**Bupropion** 100 mg po bid × 3 days then 100 mg tid Max: 450 mg/day	Depression	Cardiac dysrhythmia, hypertension, rash, weight change, constipation, nausea, dry mouth, pharyngitis, confusion, dizziness, headache, insomnia, tremor, agitation, anxiety
C	**Trazodone** 150 mg/day po in 3 divided doses Max: 400 mg/day Increase, if necessary, at intervals of ≥ 1 wk.	Often useful in combination with SSRI/SNRI in relieving insomnia	Sweating, weight change, GI disturbance, dry mouth, dizziness, headache, insomnia, memory impairment, somnolence, blurred vision
Anxiolytics			
	As per use in mood and anxiety disorders		

FETAL EFFECTS	LACTATION
Bupropion Pregnancy Registry of 354 women treated in first trimester and prospectively followed had a 3.4% rate of congenital anomalies (no specific pattern). This is not very different from the background rate.	Based on milk levels in human studies, theoretical risk of exposure for a breastfeeding infant is 2% of maternal weight-adjusted dose.
In small number of cases (>160) reported, no increased risk of fetal malformations.	Very small amount excreted into breast milk, but amount of potentially active metabolites not studied.
As a group, have a slightly higher than expected rate of malformations observed for monotherapy, but no causal relationship established for most agents in this category.	There is little available information. Avoid polypharmacy. Use the minimal effective dose. Monitor the infant closely for adverse effects.

Table 17.1 Medications: Off-label, continued

PREGNANCY CATEGORY	DRUG AND DOSAGES: INITIAL AND MAXIMUM	INDICATIONS (OFF LABEL IN PREGNANCY)	COMMON MATERNAL ADVERSE EFFECTS (>4%)
Anxiolytics			
D	**Lorazepam** 0.5–1 mg/d	Anxiety Insomnia	Sedation, dizziness, asthenia Prominent discontinuation symptoms if used regularly then stopped abruptly. Avoid in those at risk for hypoventilation (e.g., sleep apnea).
D	**Clonazepam** 0.25–1 mg/d	As above for lorazepam.	As above for lorazepam.
Antipsychotics			
C	**Quetiapine** 25 mg po qhs, titrated upwards to 200 mg	Can be useful in augmenting SSRIs in the treatment of OCD, anxiety, depression	Orthostatic hypotension, weight gain, GI disturbance, somnolence, dizziness, tardive dyskinesia (rare), neuroleptic malignant syndrome (rare)

FETAL EFFECTS	LACTATION
No evidence of teratogenicity. When used in high doses or regularly two weeks before delivery, may cause hypotonia, respiratory depression or poor suckling at birth. An unconfirmed association with anal atresia has been reported.	Small amount is excreted into the breast milk.
Regular use in combination with paroxetine has shown increased levels of paroxetine in maternal serum and a greater risk of transient neonatal withdrawal symptoms. When used in high doses or regularly two weeks before delivery, may cause hypotonia, respiratory depression or poor suckling at birth.	As above for lorazepam.
Manufacturer's registry reported 8/464 congenital malformations. Small placental transfer (only 23%). No neonatal withdrawal noted under 200 mg. Neurodevelopmental study in children (up to 3 yrs) showed no long-term effects.	Maternal doses 100 mg or less not detected in infant serum, and doses of 75 mg or less are not detectable in breast milk.

Table 17.1 Medications: Off-label, continued

PREGNANCY CATEGORY	DRUG AND DOSAGES: INITIAL AND MAXIMUM	INDICATIONS (OFF LABEL IN PREGNANCY)	COMMON MATERNAL ADVERSE EFFECTS (>4%)
Tricyclic antidepressants			
			Limited by numerous side-effects including constipation, dry mouth, weight gain, and sedation
C	**Amitriptyline** 75 mg per day divided into 1–3 doses po Max: 150 mg/day Increase, if necessary, at intervals of ≥ 1 wk.	Depression	Weight gain, bloating, constipation, dry mouth, dizziness, headache, somnolence, blurred vision, fatigue, cardiac dysrhythmia (frequency not defined), orthostatic hypotension
Monoamine oxidase inhibitors			
		Avoid use	After stopping, must allow at least 14 days prior to starting an SSRI

Read the manufacturer's information before prescribing, particularly: dosing, cautions, contraindications, monitoring and drug interactions. At least weekly contact in the first month or two of initiating pharmacotherapy is recommended to monitor course, in particular, the risk of self-harm.

FETAL EFFECTS	LACTATION
Clomipramine associated with congenital heart defects. Very small amounts in breast milk. Long-term follow-up shows no cognitive-behavioural differences in children exposed in utero.	
CNS effects, limb deformities and developmental delay have been noted in case reports but not confirmed with larger retrospective studies. Neonatal withdrawal symptoms have been described.	1.9% of the weight-adjusted maternal dose is estimated to be excreted into breast milk.
MAOIs are associated with fetal growth restriction.	

*Pregnancy category C: Either studies in animals have demonstrated adverse fetal effects or there are no controlled data from studies in women.

**Pregnancy category D: Studies in pregnant women (controlled or observational) have demonstrated a risk to the fetus.

Adjunctive measures
· Lifestyle and personal health interventions (see page 314)
· Couples counselling
· Addiction medicine
· Educational support groups

Child protection issues

· Be especially aware if there is ongoing abuse of alcohol or other drugs in the home.
· The appropriate ministry must be alerted immediately if there is any suspicion of harm, through neglect or abuse, being done to a child.
· Make every effort to establish a rapport of safety—many women are terrified of their babies being taken away from them and this feeds into their anxiety.
· Emphasize that the goal is to restore her to a position where she can care for her own child.

Pre-pregnancy consultation

· Evaluate the patient's current mood state.
· Assess carefully if depression is likely to occur in future pregnancies.
· Review treatment options based on severity and frequency.
· Discuss the possibility of medications in pregnancy.
· Assess safety on a case-by-case basis.
· Always invite the partner to participate.

References

Alwan, S., Reefhuis, J., Rasmussen, S.A., Olney, R.S., & Friedman, J.M. for the National Birth Defects Prevention Study. (2007). Use of selective serotonin-reuptake inhibitors in pregnancy and the risk of birth defects. *New England Journal of Medicine, 356* (26), 2684–2692.

Bennett, H.A., Einarson, A., Taddio, A., Koren, G. & Einarson, T.R. (2004). Prevalence of depression during pregnancy: systematic review. *Obstetrics and Gynecology, 103* (4), 698–709.

Chambers, C.D., Hernandez-Diaz, S., Van Marter, L.J., Werler, M.M., Louik, C., Kenneth Lyons Jones, K.L. et al. (2006). Selective serotonin-reuptake inhibitors and risk of persistent pulmonary hypertension of the newborn. *New England Journal of Medicine, 354* (6), 579–587.

Cox, J.L., Holden, J.M. & Sagovsky, R. (1987). Detection of postnatal depression. Development of the 10-item Edinburgh Postnatal Depression Scale. *British Journal of Psychiatry, 150*, 782–786.

GlaxoSmithKline. (2005). Paroxetine prescribing information. [Letter, December, 2005]. Retrieved from www.gsk.com/media/paroxetine/pregnancy_hcp_letter.pdf

Goodman, S.H. & Gotlib, I.H. (1999). Risk for psychopathology in the children of depressed mothers: A developmental model for understanding mechanisms of transmission. *Psychology Review, 106* (3), 458–490.

Louik, C., Lin, A.E., Werler, M.M., Hernandez-Diaz, S. & Mitchell, A.A. (2007). First-trimester use of selective serotonin-reuptake inhibitors and the risk of birth defects. *New England Journal of Medicine, 356* (26), 2675–2683.

Misri, S., Reebye, P., Kendrick, K., Carter, D., Ryan, D., Grunau, R.E. et al. (2006). Internalizing behaviors in 4-year-old children exposed in utero to psychotropic medications. *American Journal of Psychiatry, 163* (6), 1026–1032.

Moses-Kolko, E.L., Bogen, D., Perel, J., Bregar, A., Uhl, K., Levin, B. et al. (2005). Neonatal signs after late in utero exposure to serotonin reuptake inhibitors. *Journal of the American Medical Association, 293* (19), 2372–2383.

Sanz, E.J., De-las-Cuevas, C., Kiuru, A., Bate, A. & Edwards, R. (2005). Selective serotonin reuptake inhibitors in pregnant women and neonatal withdrawal syndrome: A database analysis. *Lancet, 365* (9458), 482–487.

Weissman, M.M., Pilowsky, D.J., Wickramaratne, P.J., Talati, A., Wisniewski, S.R., Fava, M., et al. for the STAR*D-Child Team. (2006). Remissions in maternal depression and child psychopathology: A STAR*D-child report. *Journal of the American Medical Association, 295* (12), 1389–1398. Erratum in: *Journal of the American Medical Association* (2006), *296* (10), 1234.

18

Parenting issues

ELLEN LIPMAN AND BRENDA MILLS*

Becoming a parent is exciting, but parenting can be challenging. While many factors influence parenting (e.g., culture, role models, physical and mental health, socioeconomic factors affecting the parent), most parents want to do the best job they can.

Parenting issues are a common concern brought to family doctors. Parenting issues and strategies vary according to the age and developmental stage of the child. However, there are some guiding principles that are applicable across ages and developmental stages.

Talk with parents about successful parenting
Building a strong relationship with the child is crucial. For that reason, primary care clinicians should be open to asking parents about parenting.

Three key questions to ask in primary care
1. "Would you like to discuss any concerns you have about parenting?"
2. "On a scale of zero to 10, how confident are you in your parenting, with zero being not confident and 10 being extremely confident?"
3. "What do you feel would be helpful in order to boost your confidence?"

*The authors thank Dr. Harriet MacMillan for content and editorial contributions.

When discussing these questions, parents should be encouraged to do the following:

- Establish a trusting relationship with the child. This requires listening to the child and providing unconditional love and nurturance.
- Become familiar with the appropriate behaviour for the child's age, and stage of development.
- Have realistic expectations of the child, based on the child's age and stage of development.
- Provide children with clear rules, limits, routines and consequences for breaking rules or defying limits. This provides a stable base that is helpful for children of all ages.
- Provide guidelines and supervision in order to allow children to feel safe and secure. Parents also need to have flexibility and openness to adjusting expectations.
- Approach discipline as something built on a foundation of respect, modelling, teaching and guiding. Discipline is not forcing obedience. Parents are the most important role models for their children.
- See communication with the child as being fundamentally important. Parents need to be aware of their tone of voice and body language, and to be clear about expectations. Parents should be encouraged to let children participate in decision making where possible, as this may make them more motivated to follow through with expectations.
- Spend time with the child. This includes all types of activities, such as playing and having fun, snuggle time, reading, going for a walk, having a snack or meal together.

Addressing behavioural issues

To promote positive behaviour and self-esteem, parents should:

- acknowledge and encourage positive behaviour because this promotes positive self-esteem in children
- look for opportunities to praise the child's behaviour
- build on the positives rather than focus on negatives
- use positive reinforcement strategies to reinforce desired behaviour (e.g., verbal praise, special time with child, earning rewards).

Dealing with problem behaviour

Behaviour is one of the primary ways that children, especially young children, express their feelings. Parents need to look beyond the behaviour to gain an understanding of how the child is feeling. For example, crying could be due to fatigue, hunger, disappointment or feeling lonely or sad.

Effective discipline does not instill shame, guilt, a sense of abandonment or a loss of trust. When dealing with problem behaviour, parents need to try to stay calm and keep their emotions in check. Parents may be more negative and harsh if they discipline when upset. It can help if parents take a moment before dealing with the problem behaviour situation. This usually means stepping away from the situation until calm and thinking about the appropriate reaction (one that will not make the situation bigger or worse).

The following are some specific strategies that parents should use:
- Emphasize the negative behaviour and not the child as being negative or bad.
- Put immediate consequences into place if possible, and connect them to the negative behaviour (e.g., if they didn't put their bike away, they lose the bike for the day; or, if they throw cereal on floor, they must pick it up).
- Prioritize the rules. It is often best to ignore little things.
- Do not dwell on the negative behaviour. Begin each day with a fresh start and a new outlook.

Addressing communication issues

COMMUNICATING WITH THE CHILD
Communication with a child is central to developing a positive relationship. Parents need to be aware of the fact that physical contact is the key method of communication with very young children. Later, language is important. Aspects of communication include tone of voice, body language, listening, acknowledging another's feelings, and the use of "I" statements (e.g., "I would like you to stop that behaviour…").

COMMUNICATING WITH PARTNER AND/OR EXTENDED FAMILY
While partners and extended family members may not have identical parenting styles, it is important for parents to identify shared principles and to support each other in their implementation. For both couples and single parents, it is also important to make their extended families and other supports aware of the family's values and parenting approaches.

COMMUNICATING WITH PRIMARY CARE PROVIDERS
Parents should be encouraged to open a dialogue with their primary care providers, allowing primary care providers to provide the most appropriate, comprehensive and consistent care during the relationship.

COMMUNICATING WITH THE SCHOOL
Parents should be in regular communication with their child's school community. Such an ongoing relationship facilitates sharing positive achievements and problem-solving around difficulties.

COMMUNICATING WITH OTHERS
Parents need to be aware of their child's social network and other individuals in their life.

Help parents to understand their parenting style
There are influences on parenting styles including parent temperament, cultural norms, values and beliefs, the parent's own upbringing, the support of and discussions with friends and family, and other influences including reading books and taking parenting classes. Offer the following practical advice to parents:
· Be flexible in your approach. Having a sense of humour can help!
· You do not have to be perfect or know all the answers. All parents have strengths and limitations. Mistakes are normal, and it is okay to ask for help.
· Make sure to take care of yourself. Be aware of key stresses in your life and how they influence your level of patience and ability to cope with upsets on a day-to-day basis.
· Learn ways to calm yourself.

· Establish good communication and consistency within your family as part of your parenting approach.

Talk with parents about "normal behaviour"

· Normal behaviour varies according to age and developmental stage.
· Each child is unique and behaviour varies according to a child's temperament.
· Children with special needs and developmental delay require additional adjustments and problem-solving. For more information, parents can be directed to *You and Your Child: Making Sense of Learning Disabilities* (Hollins & Hollins, 2005).
· Testing limits is normal child behaviour.
· Certain parenting styles are associated with more childhood behavioural problems and parent–child conflict. For example, harsh, punitive, inconsistent parenting styles including yelling, name-calling and spanking are associated with childhood aggression and may be associated with other mental health problems later in life.
· If parents are concerned that there are problems, encourage them to seek help. Early intervention before the age of eight years is associated with the best outcomes.
· It is best to suggest evidence-based programs to parents—for example, parenting programs such as The Incredible Years, the Triple P Positive Parenting Program (Sanders et al., 2002) ,and COPE for children three years of age and up (Cunningham et al., 1995).
· Parental readiness to engage in programs and other barriers (e.g., timing, travel, location, cost, language) may limit participation.
· Availability of programs varies considerably depending on geographic location, and there may be more reliance on primary care providers to screen and counsel families where there are few additional resources.
· There is a great deal of variation between Internet site reliability of information. Directing families to well-established sites is recommended (see the section on website resources below).

Tips for primary care providers

Build a relationship with families:

· Parenting is an important part of child and family health. Primary care clinicians have a unique opportunity to establish regular dialogue about parenting and its relation to overall child health as part of the ongoing comprehensive health care.

· A discussion about parenting can be made a part of the early regular well-baby and immunization visits, with a focus not just on the health of the child but also on the developing relationship between the parent and child. The opportunity to discuss parenting practices at this early stage will emphasize the importance of parenting practices across the developmental span.

How to use your time effectively when visiting with families:

· Use routine screening questionnaires to optimize your time—for example, Rourke Well-Baby Record (www.rourkebabyrecord.ca), Nipissing District Developmental Screen (www.ndds.ca), Pediatric Symptom Checklist (www.brightfutures.org/mentalhealth/pdf/professionals/ped_sympton_chklst.pdf).

· When possible, allow extra time for visits through use of allied health professionals. Take a team approach to working with families. Allied health professionals can play an important role in the discussion with parents about the importance of parenting.

Listen below the surface of questions:

· Empathizing with parenting stress and worry is an important part of validating a parent's concerns.

· Behavioural problems can be the manifestation of something more complex, and quick suggestions about behaviour management may increase the difficulties without getting at the underlying issues.

Create a family-friendly environment in your office:

· The physical environment can include magazines and other literature about parenting that parents can take with them.

- Include toys that allow interaction between parents and children across a range of developmental stages in the waiting area.
- A collaborative approach by the "team" in a primary care setting (which includes everyone who works in the office) will allow consistent emphasis on the importance of the parenting role.

Identify risk factors and behaviours:
- Parental mental health problems (e.g., maternal depression, substance abuse), parent relationship discord and socioeconomic disadvantage are established risk factors for emotional and behavioural problems in children.
- Primary care providers have a unique knowledge of the family and the opportunity to recognize and facilitate access to appropriate supports for families.
- Awareness of community resources for parents, particularly for young families, is important (e.g., Ontario Early Years Centres, public health).

Child safety

Physical and emotional safety are paramount for a child's healthy development. Unfortunately, there are times when suspicions of maltreatment need to be reported. In Ontario, to locate the Children's Aid Society in your area visit www.oacas.org or nationally through the Child Welfare League of Canada (http://www.cwlc.ca/files/file/policy/Welfare%20of%20Canadian %20Children%202007.pdf).

When is it necessary to report concerns to a Children's Aid agency?

There is often uncertainty as to when it is necessary to report a concern to Children's Aid. Current legislation requires reporting if you suspect child maltreatment. It is not the primary care provider's role to prove or verify maltreatment.

Child protection legislation is determined on a provincial basis, and the age of children to whom reporting requirements pertain may vary, but generally reporting must be done for a child less than 16 years of age. As an initial step, an inquiry call can be made anonymously to a central intake worker at your local Children's Aid agency. This will help to determine if the situation warrants reporting.

WHAT IS CONSIDERED REPORTABLE
Physical abuse
· Physical abuse involves bodily harm to a child by a caregiver. For example, this could include hitting, shaking or burning a child.

Sexual abuse
· Sexual abuse is any sexual activity with a child by a caregiver. For example, this could include fondling, sexual intercourse or exposure to sexual activity.

Emotional harm
· Emotional harm occurs when there is an absence of a nurturing environment for the child. It can also occur when the caregiver continually treats the child in a negative, demeaning manner.

Neglect
· Neglect is usually a pattern of failure to provide the child's physical needs such as food, clothing and shelter. It can also mean a failure to provide the child's emotional needs, attention and supervision.
· The publications *Child Maltreatment in Canada: Overview Paper* (Jack et al., 2006) and *Child Maltreatment: A "What to Do" Guide for Professionals Who Work with Children* (Cheng et al., 2006) were supported by the National Clearinghouse on Family Violence (www.phac-aspc.gc.ca/ncfv-cnivf/family violence/index.html) and are available for download.

Refusing to provide necessary medical treatment
· According to Ontario's *Child and Family Services Act*, Section (37) (2) (e), a child is in need of protection if:

- a child requires medical treatment to cure, prevent or alleviate physical harm or suffering and the child's parent (or person having charge of the child) does not provide or consent to the treatment.
· National guidelines can be investigated through the Child Welfare League of Canada (www.cwlc.ca/files/file/policy/Welfare%20of%20Canadian% 20Children%202007.pdf).

Online resources for families
· KidsHealth (www.kidshealth.org). An excellent website for caregivers, children and youth. Topics are practical, consumer-friendly and interactive. The Kids and Teens section is interactive, informative and humorous.
· Caring for Kids (www.caringforkids.cps.ca). Developed by the Canadian Paediatric Society with topics on child development, parenting, teen health and nutrition. A consumer-friendly website with downloadable resources.
· American Academy of Child and Adolescent Psychiatry (www.aacap.org/cs/ root/facts_for_families/facts_for_families). Facts for Families provides concise and up-to-date information on issues that affect children, teenagers and their families.
· The Incredible Years (www.incredibleyears.com). A website for the Incredible Years parenting programs.
· Triple P (www1.triplep.net). A website for the Triple P Positive Parenting Program.
· Healthy Choices in Pregnancy (www.hcip-bc.org). A resource website regarding women's health concerns related to pregnancy and substance use. Developed by the Centre of Excellence for Women's Health and BC Women's Hospital & Health Centre.

References

Cheng, C., Munn, C., Jack, S. & MacMillan, H. for the National Clearinghouse on Family Violence. (2006). *Child Maltreatment: A "What to Do" Guide for Professionals Who Work With Children*. Ottawa: Public Health Agency of Canada. Retrieved from http://www.phac-aspc.gc.ca/ncfv-cnivf/pdfs/nfnts-2006-cmt_e.pdf

Cunningham, C.E., Bremner, R. & Boyle M. (1995). Large group community-based parenting programs for families of preschoolers at risk for disruptive behaviour disorders: Utilization, cost effectiveness, and outcome. *Journal of Child Psychology Psychiatry, 36* (7), 1141–1159. DOI:10.1111/j.1469-7610.1995.tb01362.x

Jack, S., Munn, C., Cheng, C. & MacMillan, H. for the National Clearinghouse on Family Violence (2006). *Child Maltreatment in Canada: Overview Paper*. Ottawa: Public Health Agency of Canada. Retrieved from http://www.canadiancrc.com/PDFs/2006_Canadian_Child_Maltreatment_Overview_En.pdf

Hollins, S. & Hollins, M. (2005). *You and Your Child: Making Sense of Learning Disabilities*. London, England: Karnac Books.

Sanders, M.R., Turner, K.M., & Markie-Dadds, C. (2002). The development and dissemination of the Triple P Positive Parenting Program: A multilevel, evidence-based system of parenting and family support. *Prevention Science, 3* (3), 173–189.

19

Improving collaboration between mental health and primary care services

NICK KATES AND MARILYN CRAVEN

Background

Since the mid-1990s there has been rapidly increasing interest in new, more collaborative partnerships between mental health and primary care services. Providers are seeing the benefits of better collaboration between the primary care and mental health care sectors and funders are looking at ways to incorporate collaborative practice in their planning processes. These new approaches have included:

· programs that aim to improve the flow of patients between mental health and primary care services
· programs that integrate mental health services into primary care settings
· initiatives that aim to provide better physical health care for people with mental health problems
· educational programs that bring professionals from different disciplines together to learn with and from one another
· training programs that increase the familiarity, comfort and skills of future practitioners in working in new collaborative approaches
· planning activities at the federal, provincial, territorial, regional and local levels that have brought together providers from mental health and primary care settings, as well as patient and family representatives, to address common issues.

The trend toward greater collaboration between mental health and primary health services is consistent with a commitment to better collaboration at all levels of Canada's health services, and to improved systems of health care delivery. Such collaboration makes it easier for consumers to receive the services they require, from the most suitable health care provider, in the most accessible location and with a minimum of obstacles.

This chapter summarizes reasons for improving collaboration between mental health and primary care services and the principles that should guide new initiatives; outlines a number of strategies for improvement, many of which can be implemented in any clinical setting with little cost; and presents practical tips for setting up new collaborative projects, whatever their scope.

Why do we need better collaboration?

· The prevalence of mental health problems in primary care is high and increasing.
· Primary care providers play a major role in delivering mental health care in every Canadian community.
· Many mental health problems can be treated successfully in primary care settings if there is increased support to facilitate guideline-level care.
· Detection and treatment initiation rates for mental health problems in primary care remain low (Timonen & Liukkonen, 2008). Many individuals with mental health problems receive no treatment over the course of a year, even though they may see their family physician.
· Traditional mental health settings may not be able to reach many of these individuals, but primary care is more likely to be able to do so.
· Stigma remains a problem for individuals with mental health problems. When care is delivered in the primary care setting, stigma is often reduced.
· Many mental health problems are chronic and recurring, with high rates of medical comorbidity. Individuals with mental health problems are less likely to receive appropriate medical care than individuals without mental illness, particularly if they are treated only in the formal mental health system.
· Comorbid depression and anxiety often complicate the course of a general medical condition, leading to increased mortality and morbidity rates, and

these problems are rarely addressed. Primary care is the logical place to identify mental health problems and initiate treatment.
· Shortages of family physicians, psychiatrists and other specialized mental health resources make it an imperative to use existing resources as efficiently and effectively as possible. Close collaboration permits difficult, complex problems to be jointly managed, and makes better use of the skills of each member of the team.
· No single provider can be expected to have the time and skills to provide all the necessary care a patient may require — this is best achieved through collaborative partnerships and well-functioning teams.
· Better collaboration can improve access to mental health care, especially for populations that traditionally under-utilize mental health services.
· Closer collaboration between mental health services and primary care provides new opportunities for:
  - health and mental health promotion
  - illness (relapse) prevention
  - early detection and treatment of mental health problems
  - improving collegiality
  - enhancing clinical skills.

Problems between the two sectors

The potential benefits of better collaboration between primary care and the formal mental health care system are enormous, but there are many problems and obstacles to collaboration at the interface between the two sectors, including:
· Poor communication. Patients are often perceived to "disappear" into the care of the mental health system, with little information going back to the family physician during treatment. Conversely, many psychiatrists are frustrated by inadequate information at the time of referral. Delays in sending discharge or consultation notes leave family physicians frustrated and feeling unsure about their treatment.
· Difficulty with access. Family physicians often view referral processes as "bureaucratic nightmares," especially for emergency consultations.
· Lack of understanding of, or respect for, the role of the family physician.
· Lack of support for primary care providers.

Does improved collaboration improve patient outcomes?

Improved collaboration does improve patient outcomes, but analyses of the outcomes literature show that collaboration paired with treatment guidelines produces significantly better outcomes than either collaboration alone or guideline-level care alone. In addition, some patients may benefit more than others. A stepped approach to care, with more extensive collaboration targeted at patients with more severe or serious problems may help to optimize the use of treatment resources.

Principles to guide collaborative care

If a collaborative initiative is to succeed, it needs to be based on the following principles:

· Primary care and mental health services should be seen as part of a well-integrated continuum of mental health services, with minimal barriers between the sectors.

· A collaborative initiative must be relevant to the local context and culture and adapted to fit the needs of providers and patients.

· It needs to be patient-centred with patients and their families being actively involved in all aspects of service delivery.

· It should be based on an analysis of local needs, and it should build upon current strengths and existing relationships.

· Collaborative partnerships must be based on mutual respect and trust along with a recognition of each partner's potential roles and contributions.

· The roles, activities and responsibilities of different providers need to be defined, co-ordinated, complementary and responsive to the changing needs of patients, their families, other caregivers and resource availability.

· Collaborative partnerships need to have clearly identified goals and be based on what the literature has shown to be effective practices.

· New collaborative initiatives should build in an evaluation component to permit ongoing refinements in service delivery, and to ensure adequate accountability to all stakeholders.

· Collaborative practice needs to be supported by changes in health system design and funding.

Strategies to improve collaboration

While one approach to improving collaboration involves the integration and delivery of mental health services within primary care settings, there are many other ways that collaboration between the two sectors can be improved. Many of the examples listed below can be implemented with little or no additional funding.

Make psychiatric services more responsive to primary care

- Review current intake processes with primary care providers using the service, and look for ways to make them simpler and more user-friendly. Review what information is required at the initial point of contact. This review should include exclusion criteria that may make little sense to a primary care provider (such as not treating someone who has an alcohol problem and depression for his or her depression until the individual has received addiction treatment elsewhere).
- Ensure that the family physician is involved (usually by a phone call) in discharge planning and that a copy of the discharge plan is faxed to the physician on the day of discharge from inpatient or outpatient care. A copy of the plan can also be given to the patient so he or she is aware of what is involved, and can hold all parties accountable.
- Consider holding the discharge appointment in the primary care setting instead of the outpatient clinic or inpatient unit. That way everyone who is involved in the person's care can discuss the plan and their respective roles and responsibilities. This is particularly useful for complex cases involving multiple providers.
- Institute telephone back-up one or two mornings a week for primary care providers who need to speak to a psychiatrist (within the half-day) about cases or problems.
- Provide proactive follow-up. Some innovative outpatient services routinely keep a case open for six months after completing an episode of care. At three and six months they will call patients to find out how they are doing and whether they have connected with their family physician. They will also ask whether or not patients are aware of the plan for their care, if they are still taking their medications and if they are experiencing any side-effects.

If things are going well, the case is closed at six months. If things are not going well, patients can be seen again, or linkages can be facilitated and the same review process reinstituted.

· To help address wait-time challenges, mental health services can offer a rapid consultation service to primary care. A treatment plan is worked out and provided to the patient and the primary care provider. The patient will then return to the primary care setting for ongoing care and/or go back on the waiting list for ongoing treatment at the mental health clinic. Patients can also play an active role in improving communication between care providers. Give patients copies of key reports, a list of their medications and a copy of their treatment plan, and encourage them to take these with them to all medical or mental health appointments.

· Make sure reports and discharge summaries are relevant and useful. Attach brief information sheets with relevant practical advice, including the details of how to manage the medications the person is being prescribed.

· Consider developing a resource (e.g., guidebook or fact sheet) for primary care providers that lists the community resources that would be helpful in the psychiatric and psychosocial care of their patients. When developing and organizing such a resource, a problem-based rather than a service-based approach seems to work best. Entries should include at a minimum the name and address of the service, contact information for the intake worker, the programs and services offered, how a referral is made, whether there is any cost and whether there is any exclusion criteria (e.g., age, disorder).

Improve the medical care of people with a mental illness

People with mental illnesses have greater difficulty finding a primary care provider. Of those who have a primary care provider, they are less likely to have physical health problems identified than people without a mental illness. Ways to improve both access to a primary care provider and the quality of the care include:

· contracting with a local family physician(s) or nurse practitioner(s) who may be willing to visit a mental health program every one to two weeks to assess general health problems of people using that service who do not also have access to a primary care clinic

· negotiating with family physicians on an individual basis to take on more complex cases on the understanding that the mental health service will continue to provide ongoing back-up and support, even when the problems have stabilized
· ensuring that people who do have access to primary care are seen at least annually.

Increase collaboration in local planning

· Involve primary care providers in the evaluation of mental health services on a regular basis. Design an annual satisfaction survey (by mail or by phone) that also asks for suggestions for improvements that could be made. The information gathered will be helpful and family physicians will appreciate being asked, especially if their comments lead to changes in the services offered.
· Mental health and primary care providers need to be involved in each other's planning and needs analysis processes.

Increase joint educational activities

· Organize joint clinical/educational rounds for primary care and mental health providers. Such opportunities allow people not only to learn with and from each other, but also to get to know each other, have an opportunity to discuss cases informally, and make connections that will improve the flow of cases from one sector to the other.
· In academic settings, workshops/tutorials should be offered that bring together family medicine and psychiatry residents, and possibly other learners, to begin to understand what each can bring to a collaborative partnership early in their careers.

Integrate mental health services in primary care

Delivering mental health services in the primary care setting has been demonstrated to be an effective way to increase access to mental health services. It also helps to improve communication between family physicians and mental health care specialists, increase co-ordination and continuity of care, and facilitate early detection and treatment of mental health problems.

While there are many ways to deliver mental health services in primary care, one successful approach involves attaching a mental health worker (MHW) to a primary care practice. This can be done for one or more half-days a week, according to practice size, supported by a visiting psychiatrist. An ideal ratio may be one full-time MHW for every three to four family physicians, with a psychiatrist visiting for approximately half a day per month per family physician. In reality, these ratios will need to be adjusted, according to the availability of resources. In general, the less time there is available with the psychiatrist or MHW, the more time the psychiatrist or MHW should spend on consultations and assessments, with implementation of care plans being handed back to primary care clinicians. The emphasis should be on discussing patient problems and working out a plan together rather than providing assessments on everyone.

For integrated mental health care to work optimally, mental health care providers need to:
· understand the demands of primary care (the fast pace, the frequent interruptions, the unpredictability)
· be respectful of and adapt to the environment and routines of the primary care setting
· be clear about the limitations of what they are able and not able to offer
· allow time for case discussions and case reviews with the family physician, as well as seeing new patients
· make these case discussions brief and relevant, with as much practical, how-to information as possible
· chart (legibly) in the continuing medical record (electronic or paper) before leaving the office
· provide clear and concise treatment plans, with contingencies built in for failure to respond and for crises.

Family physicians and other primary care providers need to:
· attempt to find serviceable space for the mental health clinician and the visiting psychiatrist
· be willing to spend time reviewing cases, providing guidance for the mental health providers as to how and when they would like this to occur

- be willing to discuss patient problems and implement advice rather than refer everyone for a consultation from the visiting psychiatrist or the attached mental health worker
- follow through with the agreed treatment plan once care is handed back
- champion this approach with other primary care staff.

Together, the mental health and primary care providers need to:
- meet periodically to evaluate the collaborative program and make any necessary adjustments
- determine which patient populations and/or mental health care problems are the priorities for collaborative care
- work out how appointments will be made, charts pulled, notes written, reports dictated, etc.
- meet at the start of each day to review who is coming in (for the family physician and the mental health team), what their care needs may be and how, if necessary, each could help the other
- meet periodically to review how the model is working.

Setting up a collaborative care initiative

Irrespective of the nature of the project, there are some basic steps to follow with any collaborative project, if it is to succeed:
- Representatives of providers and key support personnel in the mental health and primary care settings/communities should meet early in the planning process to identify the changes they want to make and how they might do this. This may involve some preliminary "clearing the air" in identifying often long-standing issues and problems, with the agreement to discuss these, get them out of the way and move on. Planning groups should include patients in the design and evaluation whenever possible.
- Determine whether new funding is likely to be available and, if so, whether it is for a time-limited period or ongoing. If funding is not available, the challenge will be to improve services by changing existing processes or procedures. Funding sources must be identified early on, and the duration of the funding must be clear.

- Ideally start small and expand the project once it has achieved its initial goals and lessons have been learned.
- Identify a planning/monitoring group for the project. The planning group will identify:
  - the goals of the project
  - how they will know if it is succeeding
  - where to start (it is usually advisable to start with a smaller, manageable change, with the next stage of the project being influenced by what is learned from the first steps)
  - how the project will be monitored
  - how often the planning group will meet
  - what staffing or other resources may be required.
- Senior leadership in the participating services should take responsibility for ensuring that the project is "sold" to other staff and emphasize their commitment to making it work.
- The project team should meet monthly initially to look at lessons being learned and the implications for the service.

Resources
- Canadian Collaborative Mental Health Initiative website: www.ccmhi.ca
- Collaborative Mental Health Care website: www.shared-care.ca

References

Craven, M. & Bland, R. (2006). Better practices in collaborative mental health care: An analysis of the data base. *Canadian Journal of Psychiatry, 51* (Suppl. 1).

Kates, N., Craven, M., Bishop, J., Clinton, T., Kraftcheck, D., LeClair, K. et al. (1997). Shared mental health care in Canada. *Canadian Journal of Psychiatry, 42* (Suppl. 8) and *Canadian Family Physician, 43* (Suppl. Oct.). Ottawa: Canadian Psychiatric Association and College of Family Physicians of Canada.

Kates, N., Crustolo, A., Farrar, S. & Nikolaou, L. (2001). Integrating mental health services in primary care: Lessons learnt. *Families, Systems and Health, 19* (1), 5–12. DOI: 10.1037/h0089457

Kates, N. & Mach, M. (2007). Chronic disease management for depression in primary care: A summary of the current literature and implications for practice. *Canadian Journal of Psychiatry, 52* (2), 77–86.

Lester, H., Freemantle, N., Wilson, S., Sorohan, H., England, E., Griffin, C. et al. (2007). Cluster randomised controlled trial of the effectiveness of primary care mental health workers. *British Journal of General Practice, 57* (536), 196–203.

The Standing Senate Committee on Social Affairs, Science and Technology. (2006). *Out of the Shadows at Last: Transforming Mental Health, Mental Illness and Addiction Services in Canada*. Ottawa: The Senate of Canada.

Timonen M. & Liukkonen T. (2008). Management of depression in adults. *British Medical Journal, 336* (7641), 435–439. DOI: 10.1136/bmj.39478.609097.BE

Wagner, E.H., Austin, B.T., Davis, C., Hindmarsh, M., Schaefer, J. & Bonomi A. (2001). Improving chronic illness care: translating evidence into action. *Health Affairs, 20* (6), 64–78.

20

Supported self-management for common mental health problems

DAN BILSKER AND J. ELLEN ANDERSON

What is supported self-management?

Supported self-management (SSM) is a low-intensity behavioural intervention in which the patient receives a self-care tool (i.e., workbook, audiofile, DVD, or web-based material) along with support by a health care provider (Nelson & Loomis, 2005; Christensen et al., 2004). Workbooks and programs developed for mental health self-care are typically based on the principles of cognitive-behavioural therapy (CBT) (Greenberger & Padesky, 1995; Bilsker & Patersson, 2005). SSM utilizes much less clinical time than does standard CBT and is suitable for delivery at the primary care level, rather than requiring involvement of scarce mental health specialists (den Boer et al., 2004). The primary care provider's role in SSM is not to be a psychotherapist, but rather a coach who assists the patient in applying the skills of behavioural change.

As an intervention in clinical practice, SSM falls somewhere between a clinical treatment, targeting mental health symptoms, and a method of knowledge transfer, teaching the patient a set of concepts and strategies helpful in overcoming mental health problems. Most work in this area has been focused on depression, but self-management tools have also been developed for panic disorder (Antony & McCabe, 2004), health anxiety (Asmundson & Taylor, 2005), eating disorder (McCabe et al., 2003) and other mental health problems.

Why is it important to deliver this intervention?

SSM delivers a number of important benefits to primary mental health care. First, it extends the reach of the primary care clinician, allowing a form of CBT that is practical within the time constraints of primary care (Whitfield & Williams, 2003). There is pressure on primary care clinicians to offer non-pharmacological intervention — SSM is a behavioural intervention that can be feasibly incorporated into standard practice (Bilsker et al., 2007). Our research group tested its feasibility in a dissemination trial with 85 family physicians: they chose to use SSM for depression with 25 per cent of their patients with depression over a six-month period, an impressive rate of uptake (Bilsker et al., 2008).

Second, acquiring a basic level of competence in SSM does not demand extensive training. A training session as brief as one hour provides sufficient grounding for SSM to be confidently delivered — although it is true that further training and experience with this intervention allows it to be used in a more sophisticated way.

Third, several systematic reviews have shown SSM for mild range depression to be effective compared to control conditions (McKendree-Smith et al., 2003). A recent systematic review found that SSM for depression yields an effect similar in magnitude to that of standard depression treatment (Gellatly et al., 2007). However, it must be kept in mind that controlled trials of self-management mostly target individuals with mild symptomatology and are not directly comparable to standard treatment trials.

Fourth, SSM is recommended by a number of care guidelines — notably those of the U.K. National Institute for Health and Clinical Excellence

(NICE), where it is referred to as guided self-help—for common mental health problems including depression, anxiety and eating disorders (National Collaborating Center for Mental Health, 2010; McIntosh et al., 2004; National Collaborating Center for Mental Health, 2004a).

Fifth, SSM for depression provides a credible alternative to antidepressant medication in mild cases. Over-reliance on medication has been highlighted by a leading expert in primary mental health care: "Evidence suggests that patients with minor depression and adjustment disorders are frequently treated with antidepressant medications, which represents 'overuse' in the IOM [Institute of Medicine] nosology since there is little evidence of effectiveness of medication in these populations" (Katon, 2003). A similar point is made by the NICE guidelines: "Antidepressants are not recommended for the initial treatment of mild depression, because the risk–benefit ratio is poor" (National Collaborating Center for Mental Health, 2004b).

Finally, SSM has low cost to the patient or the health care system. In our dissemination trial of SSM for depression, delivery of SSM cost $15, versus an average cost of $100 for a course of antidepressant medication* (Bilsker et al., 2008; Patten et al., 2008).

What are the steps of SSM for depression or other mental health problems?

Assess

The first step is to evaluate the patient's suitability for this intervention. In addition to making a clinical judgment about the patient's readiness to take on self-management, it is necessary to determine the severity of symptomatology. In determining the appropriateness of SSM for a depressed patient, a primary care provider could rely on clinical judgment, but also might find

*Neither of these cost estimates includes the physician's time.

it helpful to administer brief scales such as the PHQ-9. The PHQ-9 categorizes depressive symptomatology as *mild, moderate* or *severe.*

· If the depression falls in the mild or low-moderate range, then SSM is appropriate as a stand-alone intervention.

· If the depression falls in the high-moderate to severe categories, then SSM may be appropriate as an adjunctive intervention, along with other treatments like antidepressant medication or CBT. Even when CBT or medication is provided, it can be helpful to engage the patient in active recovery through self-management skills. It may be that certain patients are so depressed at a particular time that they are unable to focus on learning or applying self-management skills. At the same time, it is important not to automatically accept a patient's pessimistic self-evaluation, but rather to encourage the patient to try reading through a small section of the recommended workbook.

· If a patient has achieved a significant degree of recovery through treatment, SSM may well be useful in maintaining recovery and planning to prevent relapse.

A similar approach may be applied to deciding the appropriateness of SSM for other common mental health problems.

Advise

The second step is to recommend self-management, indicating (or, better, providing) the workbook or program you endorse. Advising the patient about self-management might include explaining that self-management can be quite effective and that you will be available to provide assistance in applying the skills. Although each clinician will have a unique way of communicating the importance of self-management, here are some messages to consider (these suggestions are focused on depression, but may be readily adapted to other problems):

· "The way you are feeling is something we can work together to change. There are some ideas in this (book) that many people have found very helpful, and that have proven to be very effective in managing low mood and depression. I would be happy to work with you to help you learn some of these

Figure 20.1 Factors associated with causing or continuing a depressed state

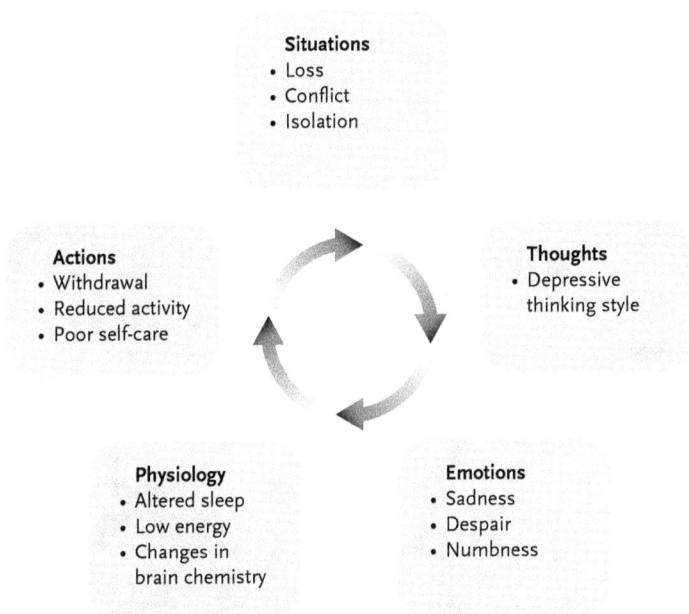

Situations
- Loss
- Conflict
- Isolation

Actions
- Withdrawal
- Reduced activity
- Poor self-care

Thoughts
- Depressive thinking style

Physiology
- Altered sleep
- Low energy
- Changes in brain chemistry

Emotions
- Sadness
- Despair
- Numbness

Reproduced with permission from Bilsker, D. & Paterson, R. (2005). *Antidepressant Skills Workbook* Vancouver: Faculty of Health Sciences, Simon Fraser University.

new approaches and ideas so you will feel better. This would require you to do a little bit of reading, some practice at home and some regular visits with me to monitor how you are doing and help you with any obstacles or problems. Does this feel like something you would like to try?"

If you are using SSM as an adjunct to other treatment, the explanation would be modified ("I recommend treatment Q—but along with Q, it would be helpful to learn some self-management skills for handling [depression] better").

A similar model for health anxiety might look like this:

Figure 20.2 Factors associated with causing or continuing an anxious state

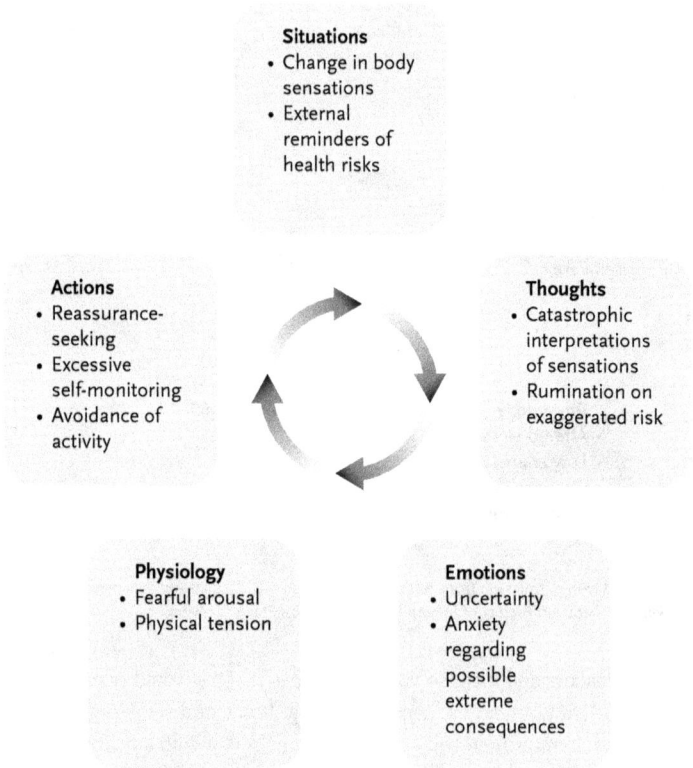

Situations
- Change in body sensations
- External reminders of health risks

Actions
- Reassurance-seeking
- Excessive self-monitoring
- Avoidance of activity

Thoughts
- Catastrophic interpretations of sensations
- Rumination on exaggerated risk

Physiology
- Fearful arousal
- Physical tension

Emotions
- Uncertainty
- Anxiety regarding possible extreme consequences

Some clinicians have adopted the approach of using a model from a self-management workbook (for example, see Figure 20.1) to show patients how mood is affected by other factors. Going over this model readily leads into a discussion of why it would be helpful to learn skills to break a cycle of negative mood. This could also be a useful way to introduce the need for other treatments.

Assist
The third step is to help your patient learn self-management skills.

HELPING THE PATIENT TO FIND A STARTING POINT
Help the patient to decide which skill to learn first, or what problem to address first. For example, if a depressed patient is inactive and socially isolated, then it might be appropriate to begin with behavioural activation (see below). If the patient is having overly negative and self-critical thoughts, then it might be appropriate to begin with cognitive restructuring (see below). Or if the patient is feeling overwhelmed by a life situation, then it might be appropriate to begin with structured problem-solving (see below).

PROVIDE ONGOING SUPPORT
Ongoing support might include encouraging the patient to keep practising the skills and assisting the patient to learn new skills and set new goals. The feasibility of providing ongoing support depends partly upon time pressures in your practice. It might only be possible for some patients, but it will make the intervention more effective.

EXPLAIN SELF-MANAGEMENT SKILLS
Although each self-management workbook or program takes a somewhat different approach and emphasizes particular skills, most will cover certain core skills. For depression, three core skills are behavioural activation, cognitive restructuring and structured problem-solving.

Behavioural activation
People who are depressed typically become less active. They withdraw from social contacts, reduce their level of self-care activities and become less active in hobbies or other activities. It may seem to the patient like a

way of conserving strength, but inactivation typically worsens the depressed mood and slows recovery. Behavioural activation is taught in a step-by-step way. Target activities are identified. Often these activities are social or self-care activities that have become less frequent with onset of depression. The patient is encouraged to make an activation plan that is:

· specific, describing in a concrete way what exactly is going to be done
· realistic, with goals that are modest and feasible even if the patient continues to feel low
· written into a schedule and crossed off when completed. Note that crossing off a completed goal may initially be the only real reward, showing the individual that he or she has met a challenge and done something useful for recovery.

Cognitive restructuring

This skill addresses the cognitive side of depression. People who are depressed often think about themselves and their situation in an unrealistically negative way. This can show up as harsh and unfair self-criticism, a pessimistic approach to the current situation and unrealistically negative expectations for the future. It can be surprising to learn the harsh thoughts depressed patients often have about themselves! To change this thinking style, the person who is depressed is shown how to identify depressive thoughts that are unrealistic, unfair and distorted. There are common depressive thinking styles. For example, people may magnify negative aspects of a situation or label themselves in a denigrating way. The person is taught to use a set of questions to identify more fair and realistic thoughts; for example, asking "can I get more evidence about the situation?" or "what would I say to a friend in the same situation?" Fair and realistic thoughts must be practised in situations where the person who is depressed would normally think in a harsh and negative manner. Each time the person notices depressive thinking, he or she must challenge the negative thoughts and practise fair and realistic alternatives.

Structured problem-solving

People who are depressed may have considerable difficulty solving problems. They tend to overestimate the severity of a problem, underestimate their own resources and feel stymied in coming up with a plan. By helping patients who are depressed to solve problems, we increase their sense of competence. This skill starts by identifying a particular problem, one that is not too difficult. Then the patient writes three actions that would at least move in the direction of solution and writes out the advantages and disadvantages of each. Finally, the patient chooses one action and starts to put it into effect. This involves making a plan that is specific, realistic and scheduled. As the patient develops problem-solving skills, more difficult problems can be addressed.

Self-management tools focused on other mental health problems will, of course, teach a different set of skills (relaxation, graduated exposure to situations, etc.).

Conclusion

Incorporating SSM into your practice is well worth consideration. It will provide you with access to a behavioural intervention that is evidence-informed and feasible to use with a substantial proportion of your patients dealing with common mental health problems. The brevity and simplicity of SSM enable you to do something valuable for patients without adding stress to your workday. If you wish to try SSM with some patients, you might begin by reading through a self-management book. For example, the Antidepressant Skills Workbook, developed by a research group at Simon Fraser University, is available for free download (see Bilsker & Paterson, 2005). We think you will find SSM to be a relevant, practical and effective tool to incorporate into your practice.

References

Antony, M. & McCabe, R.E. (2004). *10 Simple Solutions to Panic: How to Overcome Panic Attacks, Calm Physical Symptoms, & Reclaim Your Life.* Oakland, CA: New Harbinger Publications.

Asmundson, G. & Taylor, S. (2005). *It's Not All in Your Head: How Worrying about Your Health Could Be Making You Sick — and What You Can Do about It.* New York: Guilford Press.

Bilsker, D., Anderson, J., Samra, J., Goldner, E.M. & Streiner, D. (2008). Behavioural interventions in primary care: An implementation trial. *Canadian Journal of Community Mental Health, 27* (2), 179–189.

Bilsker, D. Goldner, E.M. & Jones, W. (2007). Health service patterns indicate potential benefit of Supported Self-Management for depression in primary care. *Canadian Journal of Psychiatry, 52* (2), 86–95.

Bilsker, D. & Paterson, R. (2005). *Antidepressant Skills Workbook.* Vancouver: Simon Fraser University, Centre for Applied Research in Mental Health and Addiction. Retrieved from www.comh.ca/selfcare/

Christensen, H., Griffiths, K.M. & Jorm, A.F. (2004). Delivering interventions for depression by using the internet: Randomised controlled trial. *British Medical Journal, 328* (7434), 265. DOI: 10.1136/bmj.37945.566632.EE

den Boer, P.C., Wiersma, D. & Van den Bosch, R.J. (2004). Why is self-help neglected in the treatment of emotional disorders? A meta-analysis. *Psychological Medicine, 34* (6), 959–971. DOI: 10.1017/S003329170300179X

Gellatly, J., Bower, P., Hennessy, S., Richards, D., Gilbody, S. & Lovell, K. (2007). What makes self-help interventions effective in the management of depressive symptoms? Meta-analysis and meta-regression. *Psychological Medicine, 37* (9), 1217–1228. DOI:10.1017/S0033291707000062

Greenberger, D. & Padesky, C.A. (1995). *Mind Over Mood: Change How You Feel by Changing the Way You Think*. New York: Guilford Publications.

Katon, W.J. (2003). The Institute of Medicine "Chasm" report: Implications for depression collaborative care models. *General Hospital Psychiatry, 25* (4), 222–229. DOI: 10.1016/S0163-8343(03)00064-1

McCabe, R.E., Olmsted, M.P. & McFarlane, T.L. (2003). *Overcoming Bulimia Workbook: Your Comprehensive, Step-By-Step Guide to Recovery*. Oakland, CA: New Harbinger Publications.

McIntosh, A., Cohen, A., Turnbull, N., Esmonde, L., Dennis, P., Eatock, J. et al. (2004). *Clinical Guidelines and Evidence Review for Panic Disorder and Generalised Anxiety Disorder* (Clinical Guideline 22). Sheffield: University of Sheffield/London: National Collaborating Centre for Primary Care. Retrieved from http://guidance.nice.org.uk/CG22

McKendree-Smith, N.L., Floyd, M. & Scogin, F.R. (2003). Self-administered treatments for depression: A review. *Journal of Clinical Psychology, 59* (3), 275–288.

National Collaborating Center for Mental Health. (2004a). *Eating Disorders: Core Interventions in the Treatment and Management of Anorexia Nervosa, Bulimia Nervosa and Related Eating Disorders* (Clinical Guideline 9). London, England: National Institute for Health and Clinical Excellence. Retrieved from http://www.nice.org.uk/guidance/CG9.

National Collaborating Center for Mental Health. (2004b). *Management of Depression in Primary and Secondary Care* (Clinical Guideline 23). London, England: National Institute for Health and Clinical Excellence. Retrieved from http://www.nice.org.uk/guidance/CG23/niceguidance.

National Collaborating Center for Mental Health. (2010). *Depression: The NICE Guidelines on the Treatment and Management of Depression in Adults, Updated Edition* (Clinical Guideline 90). London, England: The British Psychological Society & The Royal College of Psychiatrists. Retrieved from http://guidance.nice.org.uk/CG90.

Nelson, G. & Loomis, C. (2005). Review: Self-help interventions improve anxiety and mood disorders. *Evidence Based Mental Health, 8* (2), 44. DOI: 10.1136/ebmh.8.2.44

Patten, S.B., Williams, J.V.A. & Mitton, C. (2008). Costs associated with mood and anxiety disorders, as evaluated by telephone survey. *Chronic Diseases in Canada, 28* (4), 155–162. Retrieved from http://www.phac-aspc.gc.ca/publicat/cdic-mcc/28-4/index-eng.php

Whitfield, G. & Williams, C. (2003). The evidence base for CBT in depression: Delivering CBT in busy clinical settings. *Advances in Psychiatric Treatment, 9* (1), 21–30.

Appendix

Links to televideo shared care and telepsychiatry

This is a province-by-province scan of services, by no means comprehensive.

Yukon

YUKON TELEHEALTH NETWORK (YTN)
http://www.hss.gov.yk.ca/telehealth.php

Northwest Territories

TELEMENTALHEALTH
www.yhssa.org/clientservices/Telehealth.asp

British Columbia

BRITISH COLUMBIA MINISTRY OF HEALTH EHEALTH
www.health.gov.bc.ca/ehealth/telehealth_project.html

Alberta

ALBERTA FIRST NATIONS TELEHEALTH PROGRAM
Telephone: 780 495-4949, Fax: 780 495-8920

ALBERTA TELEHEALTH
www.health.alberta.ca/initiatives/telehealth.html

Manitoba

MB TELEHEALTH
www.mbtelehealth.ca/

Saskatchewan

TELEHEALTH SASKATCHEWAN
www.health.gov.sk.ca/telehealth

Ontario

THE ONTARIO PSYCHIATRIC OUTREACH PROGRAM
www.opop.ca/english/view.asp?x=1

Quebec

RUIS, MCGILL FACULTY OF MEDICINE:TELEHEALTH
www.medicine.mcgill.ca/ruis/Telesante_welcome.htm

Nova Scotia

NOVA SCOTIA TELEHEALTH NETWORK
www.gov.ns.ca/health/telehealth/

Nunavut

TELEHEALTH
www.ohsni.com/index.php?url=/content_pages/v/~Telehealth

New Brunswick

www.gnb.ca/0217/tele-care-e.asp

Newfoundland and Labrador

CENTRE FOR HEALTH INFORMATION: TELEHEALTH
www.nlchi.nf.ca/health_telehealth.php

Prince Edward Island

HEALTH P.E.I.
www.healthpei.ca/index.php3?number=1020498&lang=E

Index

F

The Editors

David S. Goldbloom, MD, FRCPC, is a psychiatrist and senior medical advisor, Education and Public Affairs, at CAMH. He is also a professor of psychiatry at the University of Toronto, a Distinguished Fellow of the American Psychiatric Association, a Fellow of the Canadian Psychiatric Association and board member and vice-chair of the Mental Health Commission of Canada. In 2010, CAMH published a revised first edition of Dr. Goldbloom's *Psychiatric Clinical Skills*, the essential guide to interviewing and assessing people with psychiatric disorders.

Jon Davine, MD, CCFP, FRCPC, is an associate professor in the Department of Psychiatry and Behavioural Neurosciences at McMaster University, with a cross appointment in the Department of Family Medicine. His outpatient psychiatry practice focuses on liaising with primary care physicians in the shared care model. Dr. Davine also teaches courses in behavioural sciences to family medicine residents and to family doctors in the community and has lectured nationally and internationally on this topic. He is a past Chair of the Council of Psychiatric Continuing Education (COPCE), which is affiliated with the Canadian Psychiatric Association.

www.ingramcontent.com/pod-product-compliance
Lightning Source LLC
Chambersburg PA
CBHW071829270326
41929CB00013B/1935